Interpersonal Relations in Nursing

A Conceptual Frame of Reference for Psychodynamic Nursing

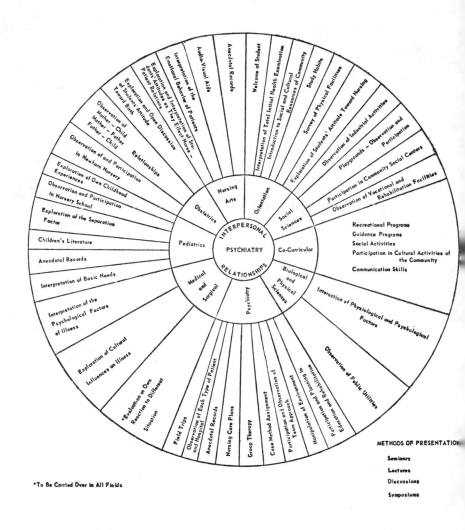

Wheel diagram labels (reading clockwise from top):

Anecdotal Records
Audio-Visual Aids
Interpretation and Open Discussion of Students' Attitude Toward Birth
Exploration and Interpretation of Students' Attitudes and Patient Relations
Interpretation of the Emotional Behavior of Patients
Observation of Mother – Child, Mother – Father, Father – Child Relationships
Observation of and Participation In Newborn Nursery
Exploration of Own Childhood Experiences
Observation and Participation In Nursery School
Exploration of the Separation Factor
Children's Literature
Anecdotal Records
Interpretation of Basic Needs
Interpretation of the Psychological Factors of Illness
Exploration of Cultural Influences on Illness
*Evaluation or Own Reaction to Different Situation
Field Trips
Observation of Each Type of Patient and Hospital
Anecdotal Records
Nursing Care Plans
Group Therapy
Case Method Assignment
Participation and Observation of Team Approach
Manipulation and Planning of Environment
Participation and Rehabilitation In Education and Rehabilitation
Observation of Public Utilities
Interaction of Physiological and Psychological Factors

Welcome of Student
Interpretation of Total Initial Health Examination
Introduction to Social and Cultural Resources of Community
Survey of Physical Facilities
Study Habits
Exploration of Students' Attitude Toward Nursing
Observation of Industrial Activities
Playgrounds – Observation and Participation
Participation in Community Social Centers
Observation of Vocational and Rehabilitation Facilities

Recreational Programs
Guidance Programs
Social Activities
Participation in Cultural Activities of the Community
Communication Skills

Inner ring: Nursing Arts, Obstetrics, Pediatrics, Medical and Surgical, Psychiatry, Biological and Physical Sciences, Co-Curricular, Social Sciences, Orientation

Center: INTERPERSONAL PSYCHIATRY RELATIONSHIPS

METHODS OF PRESENTATION

Seminars
Lectures
Discussions
Symposiums

*To Be Carried Over In All Fields

INTERPERSONAL RELATIONS IN THE
BASIC CURRICULUM

Interpersonal Relations in Nursing

A Conceptual Frame of Reference
for Psychodynamic Nursing

Hildegard E. Peplau, RN, BA, MA, EdD

Springer Publishing Company

New York

Springer Publishing Company, Inc.
536 Broadway
New York, NY 10012

91 92 93 94   /   6   5   4   3   2   1

Library of Congress Cataloging in Publication Data

Peplau, Hildegard E.
    Interpersonal relations in nursing : a conceptual frame of reference for psychodynamic nursing / by Hildegard E. Peplau
    p.   cm.
    Reprint. Originally published: Houndmills, Basingstoke, Hampshire Macmillan, 1988.
    Includes bibliographical references and index.
    ISBN 0-8261-7910-X
    1. Nurse and patient. 2. Interpersonal relations.   I. Title.
    [DNLM: 1. Nurse-Patient Relations.   2. Nursing Care—psychology
WY 87 P4221 1988a]
RT86.P4   1991
610.73'069'9—dc20
DNLM/DLC
for Library of Congress   91-4846
                                                     CIP

Printed in the United States of America

Preface

ALL books reflect, in some degree, prevailing or emerging trends coincident with the era in which they were written. This book, originally published in 1952, is no exception to that point. It considered concerns of the nursing profession in the 1950s and presented content intended to contribute toward their resolution. For instance, the question then being debated was "What is nursing?", which led to a definition of nursing as an interpersonal, investigative, nurturing, and growth-provoking process. Nursing was then viewed primarily as an art; this book presented some scientific aspects of nursing, such as theory with applications in nursing practice. A prevailing interest then was to define nursing activities in response to the question "What do nurses do?" This book shifted the question to "What do nurses know?", and focused on clinical nursing problems, concepts to explain observations, and principles to guide nurses in their work.

In writing this book, I believed that theories of interpersonal relations, then a new perspective on human interaction, were especially relevant to the work of nurses. This theoretical framework suggests that interaction phenomena that occur during nurse–patient relationships have qualitative impact on outcomes for patients. The principles and concepts introduced in this book are easily and beneficially applied in nursing practice. The concepts are basic ones—such as needs and anxiety—that provide a foundation for understanding more complex, related knowledge. In knowing and applying theory in order to understand the problems which patients present and to guide nursing interventions, nurses are adding a scientific component to the age-old arts of nursing.

In the past four decades, interpersonal theory has been greatly expanded by nursing research and by developments in the social sciences. Enrichment has also derived from such sources as theories of cognitive development and general systems theory. In other publications, I also have enlarged on the ideas presented in this original work. Nurse scholars, researchers, and clinical specialists in nursing, who found the 1952 book a starting point, have pursued empirical studies and otherwise expanded the interpersonal perspective in nursing practice. But this book remains a useful foundation in interpersonal relations theory for nurses.

H.E.P.

Professor Emerita, Rutgers University, September 1987

Foreword

THE other day I was talking with some students and members of the faculty in the Royal College of Nursing's Institute of Advanced Nursing Education in London. One said that she prized an illicit photocopy (from our Library in the RCN) of Peplau's *Interpersonal Relations in Nursing*. When I gave them the news that the book was to be republished I found myself wishing that Hildegard could have heard their whoops of joy.

This book will be received with delight by all nurses in the UK and, I believe, in so many countries of the world, as it is such an important event in the world of nursing literature.

The real reason why I believe nurses will welcome this book is that nursing in many parts of the world has lost its way with regard to the fundamentality of the nurse–patient relationship. Peplau's text and philosophy (yes—I use the word quite deliberately because I think she is truly a nursing philosopher) is clear and helpful and speaks a language which nurses want and need. We have concentrated in the last decade or so on the service of nursing—vitally important and necessary to continue so doing—but Peplau's mission is to concern herself with the art of nursing in order that it might complement and enable the service.

This book has well and truly stood the test of time, and from being described in the original Foreword as "one of the many beginning steps in studying and understanding interpersonal relations in nursing", it is now a vitally important leading work in this whole area. It is as fresh and necessary (no, more so) as the day it was written. But what changes there have been in the climate of care service since it was written. Then, patients with elective surgical conditions stayed in hospital for 10–14 days—now they stay for 10–14 hours. Then, the hospital was all—now it is only a part of the system, with people demanding more and more to be cared for in their own homes. Then, the emphasis was almost entirely on sickness, but now it is on health. These changes make the book all the more necessary and welcome. It will be used by nurses caring for the sick but it will be an exciting new discovery for nurses engaged in primary health care.

It is a privilege to have been asked by Hildegard Peplau to associate myself with this book and I do so wholeheartedly.

September 1987   Trevor Clay, MPhil, RGN, RMN, FRCN
General Secretary
The Royal College of Nursing
of the United Kingdom

Introduction

THERE IS nothing new about the kind of nursing advocated in this work. Good nurses everywhere have in varying degrees been practicing it. The purpose of this text is to aid graduate nurses and nursing students to improve their relations with patients. Many nurse practitioners wish to deepen their understanding of interpersonal relations in nursing situations in order that their work will be more effective and socially useful. Clinical instructors seek new ways for helping nursing students to develop and improve their skill in interpersonal relations. Students look for books that summarize principles that are portrayed or symbolized in the behavior of nurses who are useful to patients. This work identifies for nursing some of the concepts and principles that underlie interpersonal relations and transform nursing situations into learning experiences. It provides a reference source of hypotheses that may be examined with profit in all nursing situations. It proposes concepts that may be learned and become incorporated into the functioning personality of every nurse who is willing to struggle toward greater maturity in her relations with others.

The expression "psychodynamic nursing" is of recent origin. Spelling out the accompanying psychiatric nursing skills —their use, meaning, and consequences in general nursing— represents a more recent trend. Recognizing, clarifying, and building an understanding of what happens when a nurse relates herself helpfully to a patient are the important steps in psychodynamic nursing; nursing is helpful when both the patient and the nurse grow as a result of the learning that occurs in the nursing situation. These steps develop from the guiding assumption: *the kind of person each nurse becomes makes a substantial difference to what each patient will learn as he is nursed throughout his experience with illness.* Concepts, principles, skills, and abilities can be said to be learned when new behavior follows examination and discussion of problems that require particular principles and skills for their solution. Thus, a second guiding assumption can be stated: *fostering personality development in the direction of maturity is a function of nursing and nursing education; it requires the use of principles and methods that permit and guide the process of grappling with everyday interpersonal problems or difficulties.*

These two assumptions underlie this present work. The central task of the basic professional school of nursing is viewed as the fullest development of the nurse as a person who is aware of how she functions in a situation. A problem-attacking or problem-solving method is viewed as one of the more important ways through which this task can be met. It allows the liberation and reinforcement of ongoing processes in individual nurses and in groups. It requires attention to the unfinished tasks of earlier personality development in each student, as well as learning of skills and methods that are likely to ensure continuing forward movement. What each nurse becomes—as a functioning personality—determines the manner in which she will perform in each interpersonal contact in every nursing situation. The extent to which each nurse understands her own functioning will determine the extent to which she can come to understand the situation confronting the patient and the way he sees it. Positive, useful nursing actions flow out of understanding of the situation. Release of human interest in others who are in difficulty, liberation of emotional and intellectual capacity for making choices, development of nurses as persons whose enlightened self-interest will lead to no other choice but productive relations with all kinds of patients, students, citizens

—these are tasks related to the central one stated above. The basic task of the school of nursing ought not to be "concern for the patient", which is the task of nursing service; the task of the school of nursing is the gradual development of each nurse as a person who *wants* to nurse patients in a helpful way. Attention to this task is a guarantee of useful improvement in nursing practice.

This book is written with a view to aiding nurses and professional school personnel to recognize the importance of the nurse's personality in interpersonal relations in nursing situations. It identifies concepts and principles relevant to the promotion of psychodynamic nursing and to the resolution of interpersonal difficulties in clinical and other situations. It assumes that every nurse–patient relationship is an interpersonal situation in which recurring difficulties of everyday living arise. It recognizes that every nurse–nurse relationship is an opportunity for tackling collaboratively those disagreements in point of view that are inevitable. It takes for granted that every instructor–student relationship is an experience in interpersonal relations that becomes problematic at one time or another. Every administrator–staff nurse relationship is an interpersonal situation that calls out older feelings, unsolved difficulties, and often re-enacts problems generated in prior relationships. In every contact with another human being there is the possibility for the nurse of working toward common understandings and goals; every contact between two human beings involves the possibility of clash of feelings, beliefs, ways of acting. In nursing situations professional personnel have the obligation and the necessity to use their greater skill. Being able to understand one's own behavior, to help others to identify felt difficulties, and to apply principles of human relations to the problems that arise at all levels of experience—these are functions of psychodynamic nursing. Helping nurses to understand the relationship of nurse personalities to these functions is an aim of this work.

The day is long past when any one clinical instructor can be expected to know all of the problems and all of the principles connected with one field of work. Every instructor elects and continues to expand that which has come to her attention as relevant to nursing. Likewise, this work represents a selection of hypotheses and ideas from many sources— a selection that seemed to the author to represent basic concepts consistent with the behavior of nurses who are relatively skilful in interpersonal relations. Since it is not intended that any nurse shall limit herself to the scope of this book, references are suggested that will permit further exploration. The social sciences and psychiatry will continue to expound new ideas of importance in the solution of common nursing problems that recur in varied nursing situations.

Difficulties in human relations are not usually solved once and for all. Nor can all of the problems that we now face be fully understood in terms of ideas currently available. Nursing, as an applied science, is in a unique position to identify and study the scope, range, and varying intensities of recurring human problems that have to be faced in everyday living. Moreover, nurses help patients to meet problems at times when they are undergoing additional stresses and strains. Nurses are also in a position to identify and study degrees of skill that people use in struggling with presenting difficulties and to develop with patients the kinds of new experiences that are needed for such skill improvement. Assistance in the identification of problematic situations, appreciation and liberation of positive forces in patient personalities are functions of the nurse. As each nurse helps a patient to identify problematic elements in his current situation and to discover and understand something about what is happening to him during his illness, she *both* expands her own insights and helps the patient to grow. Thus, the nurse in some degree enables the patient to appreciate the same principles that she makes use of as she exemplifies a helping person to one in need.

Difficulties in interpersonal relations recur in varying intensities throughout the life of everyone. Sometimes the degree of skill is greater at a later date; sometimes individuals meet adult versions of an infant problem with infantile skills. The problems related to dependence provide an example: being dependent upon others is a problem that begins in infancy, changes its intensity and mode of expression as one proceeds from infancy, through adolescence, adulthood, and old age; the need can become problematic at any point in life and is the same need as seen in the infant. Only the skill with which the difficulty is evaluated and met changes as personality develops, is modified, and functions in changing situations. Each nurse should be able to identify human problems that confront patients, the degrees of skill used to meet situations, and be able to develop with patients the kind of relationships that will be conducive to improvement in skill.

Recurring difficulties can be met with greater skill at some future date, by each patient and each nurse, only when current interpersonal relations are characterized by useful learning. School of Nursing personnel provide the training ground for student nurses. The *method* by which each clinical instructor aids her trainees, basic students, to define problems and to discover and use principles in order to understand and resolve difficulties is the method that will most likely be learned. If it is exemplary of the one to be used in the nurse–patient relationship, the method will be transferred from the nursing laboratory to the clinical situation. If one method is used in the classroom and an entirely different kind is advocated for interpersonal relations in the sickroom, the student nurse is likely to be confused about the methods involved in a concept of "nurse."

Each clinical instructor, as well as every graduate nurse who has contact with students, stands for and exemplifies the meaning of the nurse concept. Whatever interpersonal relations are developed with students will, to a considerable extent, influence the concept of nursing that these students will learn. When the instructor or supervisor stands for a person who grapples with problems, inquires into new resources in order to understand the difficulty, and functions democratically with others, these qualities will tend to be evoked in students. To a marked degree students will relate to patients in the manner in which significant others (other individuals significant to them in their early life) have related to them. The patterning of student behavior may be relatively simple, clinical instructors merely reinforcing patterns already learned in parental contacts and in relations with teachers met in the past. Where the clinical instructor represents a clearly new pattern—and *mature democratic behavior is all too frequently a new pattern to be learned*—the student's wish to become like the instructor may generate difficulties, and reinforcement of earlier patterns may be impossible. When the clinical instructor's pattern of relations with students is largely a productive one she will be able to aid those students in continuing the forward struggle, in managing their frustrations, conflicts, and anxieties as older patterns of behavior are foregone and more productive, new ones are developed. As students experience this kind of useful assistance, in an interpersonal situation that is characterized by expansion of personality and productive learning, enough is learned about the method so that initially interest can develop. Deepening student understanding of the processes through which help is offered to others begins with the instructor–student relationship.

Whatever is experienced by basic students in their relations with graduate nurses in a professional program helps to pattern the behavior that will operate when they, in turn, become practicing graduate nurses. In order to understand the limitations of current practitioners it is necessary to look at the learning experiences that helped lay down patterns of present behavior. In order to recognize the kinds of patterns that are considered desirable for graduate nurse practitioners it is necessary to look at nursing situations and to find out what are the tasks or performances that are demanded of nurses; that is, *not* the activities of nurses now practicing but the *tasks* that emerge in a nurse–patient relationship. What kinds of tasks do patients present to nurses? What are the psychological demands that patients make in the presence of professional persons? How shall these demands be met so that personality of patient and nurse can be strengthened? What are the principles that govern the ways in which nurses might respond to these psychological tasks? These are questions that provide a basis for identifying the functions of psychodynamic nursing. Understanding what is involved in nurse–patient relationships is the only basis on which learning experiences for student nurses, who will develop skill in being helpful in interpersonal situations, can be designed.

While the basic school can do much to foster the development of students as useful, productive persons, each graduate nurse can also take on the responsibility for expanding her own insight into the effects of life experiences on personality functioning and for planning steps that will lead to a mode of life that is more creative and more productive. If this text proves to be helpful in an exploration of the conceptual framework and the identification of method that assists in this self-enlightenment, it will have served the useful purpose for which it has been written.

Contents

Part III. Psychological Tasks

Part IV. Methods for Studying Nursing as an Interpersonal Process

Illustrations

Part I. PHASES AND ROLES IN NURSING SITUATIONS

Purpose: *The purpose of Part I is to identify the over-all framework, to develop a whole impression with the reader about a nursing situation. This framework will then provide the structure within which influences, tasks, and methods that enter into nurse-patient relationships can be presented. Nursing, as the word is used in this work, is defined and the nursing process is viewed from the standpoint of its phases and some of the roles demanded of nurses. While clinical situations are stressed, any nurse can apply principles that are presented in any other interpersonal relationship in any area of living.*

CHAPTER I

A Definition of Nursing

Overview

EVERY NURSE practitioner has in mind a series of thoughts that expresses what she thinks nursing is about. Many nurses have put ideas on paper as definitions of nursing. Others have felt that it was not important to spend time stating what nursing is. Since this book is meant to provide a framework of concepts that are held to be basic to psychodynamic nursing, it is necessary that the author's view on nursing be included. The purpose of this chapter is to provide discussion that will contribute to an understanding of the concept of nursing, as it applies to ideas presented in later chapters and to their application in providing services to people.

Essential questions

Many questions that are necessary to making a clear definition of nursing can be raised. Considering the questions as vital to the preparation of a statement is an aspect of a problems approach, the method of procedure used in this work. The kinds of questions raised determine the scope of the investigation into the problem. Selected questions that shed light on the meaning of the concept nursing are as follows:

What is nursing? Who performs it? In what kinds of situations is it found to be useful? What can nursing do for people? How does it do what it does? When do people require nursing? Does nursing accomplish anything as an isolated function, or does it require co-operation of others? How do people go about using nursing? In general, these are the essential questions. Many accessory ones can be raised. Exploration of all queries that arise when the meaning of the word nursing is sought help the individual to get a clear picture of what is involved.

The word nursing is a symbol. As such, it stands for something more general and for something more concrete than the seven letters that appear in it. (See Fig. 1, p. 5.) The value in discussing the meaning of the word in any group is to encourage sharing of ideas, or generalizations, and thus to clarify, expand, and deepen what is meant by the concept. Examination by a group also develops consensus on the concrete actions or operations actually used by nurses as well as new ones indicated in the meaning of the word itself. Nursing practices can be designed to bring the references or preconceptions that people have about nursing more nearly in line with what the profession decides is desirable nursing action, based upon study of what is required of a nurse in nursing situations. Discussion of questions raised in defining nursing develops understanding out of which flows effective practice.

Discussion of questions

What is nursing? This is a question every student nurse needs to raise so that she becomes aware of what she feels is involved. Many take it for granted that nursing is what it now does. Haphazard development of a concept that defines a lifework and intelligent inquiry into many interrelated facets of nursing are two alternative courses of action. Inquiry points to the fact that nursing is not only what it does but what it can and ought to be doing. It sheds new light on new possibilities for service. It provides opportunity for the nursing profession to take positive steps toward bringing the references in the minds of nurses and the public more nearly in line with the referrents that grow out of nursing functions.

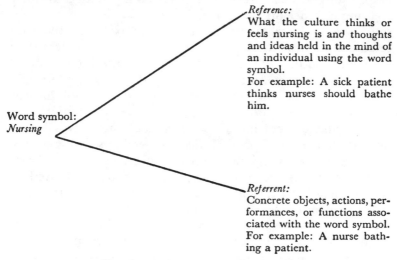

Reference:
What the culture thinks or feels nursing is and thoughts and ideas held in the mind of an individual using the word symbol.
For example: A sick patient thinks nurses should bathe him.

Word symbol:
Nursing

Referrent:
Concrete objects, actions, performances, or functions associated with the word symbol.
For example: A nurse bathing a patient.

Fig. 1.   Aspects of word symbols.

When we try to say what nursing is a number of words can be chosen that seem to symbolize and signify what is meant. It is a process, first of all. By this we mean that its serial and goal-directed nature demands certain steps, actions, operations, or performances that occur between the individual who does the nursing and the person who is nursed. Carried a step further, it may be asked: What kind of a process is nursing? Reflecting on situations in which it is needed or used, it can easily be seen that it is an *interpersonal* process and often a *therapeutic* one. This is to say that it consists in actions that require participation between two or more people and that sometimes they benefit from such interaction. Some may say, "But, some of the actions of nurses are more technical?" It can be pointed out that *the operations involved in the nursing process are interpersonal and technical ones,* but that the process itself cannot be defined as technical.

Nursing is a human relationship between an individual

who is sick, or in need of health services, and a nurse especially educated to recognize and to respond to the need for help. Interpersonal interactions between a patient and nurse —either as a person recognized in her own right or as a personification of an earlier figure in the patient's life—are often more telling in the outcome of a patient's problem than are many routine technical procedures. In the interaction of patient and nurse effort is first directed toward understanding the problem; the conditions required for resolving the difficulty may or may not include the use of technical procedures and devices but these in and of themselves would not aid the patient to grow. Indeed, procedures that are often expected to be life-saving, such as the giving of scra, intravenous infusions, etc., occasionally fail to produce desired results even when expectations of their effectiveness are high.

What is meant by the "serial and goal-directed nature" of nursing? The goals of nursing are currently in transition; its major concerns fifty years ago had to do with getting sick people well; today, nursing is more concerned with ways for helping people to stay well. Health has always been the primary goal. However, curative methods in nursing have tended to supersede development of preventive ones, but present goals include widening the sphere in which nursing offers preventive and remedial health services. Orderly steps are required for achievement of goals in any situation. A series of actions define the nursing process as it operates in various situations.

"But," many readers will assert, "nursing does not operate without medical authority." Nursing in any situation would not have full legal authority for diagnosis or treatment or all of the skills that are required by the problem to be faced. *The nursing profession has legal responsibility for the effective use of nursing and for its consequences to patients. Nursing is a function.* It is one of the many functions of a *professional health team.*[1] The authority and direction for designing nurs-

[1] The Committee on the Function of Nursing, *A Program for the Nursing Profession* (New York, The Macmillan Company, 1948), ch. V, p. 65, offers a useful definition of the word team.

ing functions derive from situations in which professional workers collaborate to bring about health improvement. Any problem to be faced by an individual or a community suggests what is needed for its solution; health workers assess problematic situations and co-operate with individuals and communities in getting needed help. Inaccurate assessment of a problem—by any professional worker—leads to functioning that may be ineffective. On the strength of retrospective analysis of difficulties that have already been met, in other situations, health educators of many kinds may foresee problems that might arise or areas in which difficulties are likely to be encountered on the basis of various kinds of evidence. Out of such experiences nursing participates in enterprises that offer preventive and remedial health services. It functions with other professional services to promote as well as to restore health in individuals and communities.

Nurses participate in delineating the many roles they can helpfully fulfill, in relation to people and to the functions of other workers in particular situations—physicians, dentists, dietitians, physiotherapists, social workers, psychologists, occupational therapists, members of the clergy, and others. Their insights are dependent upon knowledge about people, as seen in clinical and other situations, and upon the application of nursing theory and principles from all of the related science. Education and practice, close and continuous contact with patients, families, and communities make it possible for nurses to state nursing functions on the basis of some logical rationale, and to work with others in planning and carrying them out.

Professional teams organize to design plans for ensuring possible solutions to health problems of patients and communities. Nursing plans are one aspect of the total plans of a team. Professional workers also collaborate in order to encourage growth for each participating member. A team nourishes its own members so that their interrelated functions become more meaningful to each other and to the patient and the community served.

It has been pointed out that nursing is a process that is directed by a goal and that requires a series of operations in the achievement of health, for particular individuals or situations. It has also been stated that nursing is a function. Nursing is also a maturing force, and an educative instrument. By means of effective nursing, individuals and communities can be aided to use their capacities to bring about changes that influence living in desirable ways. Through contact with hospital and public health nurses, many individuals have learned new modes of responding to health problems. Slowly, individuals have learned to live comfortably and productively with disabilities such as diabetes, heart disease, deformities, and the like. Much patient teaching by nurses has encouraged mothers to bring their children to child care clinics where they could learn new ways to raise children to meet today's problems constructively. Nursing can do more than it is now doing to help people to develop and become more skillful in meeting difficulties.

When the nursing process is thought of as a maturing, educating instrument nurses develop experiences that promote constructive learning. The line between education and therapy is becoming much thinner than it was perceived to be twenty years ago. Nursing functions are both educative and therapeutic when they lead people to develop skills for solving problems. Difficulties in living recur. Problems relating to health are never solved once and for all. Solving an emergent difficulty has value but unless the individual also learns how to meet the same or a similar difficulty when it arises again, the experience has not taken the individual another step toward greater maturity in living with people.

Symonds considers therapy as a relationship that provides satisfaction for needs unmet in the past, through which continuing growth becomes possible.[2] Needs unmet in the past are often revived or intensified during illness. Physical as well as psychological needs of people—for the satisfaction of

[2] Percival Symonds, *The Dynamics of Human Adjustment* (New York, Appleton-Century-Crofts, Inc., 1946), p. 44.

their wants for food, rest, sleep, comfort, companionship, understanding—determine to considerable extent the tasks that arise in nursing situations. Can nursing meet needs that arise in ways that promote growth? [3] Are there other more deeply felt needs that arise in nurse-patient contacts? Can we say that the interpersonal nursing process is therapeutic when needs are met in a way that refreshes and restores the patient for meeting new problems? Since the nursing process has never been systematically studied from this standpoint, to find out what can or does happen when a nurse skillfully interprets and meets psychological needs we can only speculate that Symonds' hypothesis is probably true in nursing situations.

There is need to examine nursing and to find out: What can nursing do as a therapeutic, educative process? To what extent can nursing become a relationship with others that develops the personality of the nurse and the patient? One of the issues these questions raise is: shall a nurse do things *for* a patient or can participant relationships be emphasized so that a nurse comes to do things *with* a patient, as her share of an agenda of work to be accomplished in reaching a goal —health. It is likely that *the nursing process is educative and therapeutic when nurse and patient can come to know and to respect each other, as persons who are alike, and yet, different, as persons who share in the solution of problems.*

This principle needs to be examined closely, as does any basic idea that guides actions. In general, personal relationships with patients have been tabooed in nursing. Perhaps one reason for this injuction has been misunderstanding of what is a personal relationship. For purposes of nursing practice, a personal relationship is one in which two persons come to know one another well enough to face the problem at hand in a co-operative way. The relationship of nurse to patient can be represented on a continuum; at one end are two in-

---

[3] Charlotte Green Schwartz, Morris S. Schwartz, and Alfred H. Stanton, "A Study of Need-Fulfillment on a Mental Hospital Ward," *Psychiatry, Journal for the Study of Interpersonal Processes,* Vol. 14, No. 2 (May, 1951), pp. 223-42.

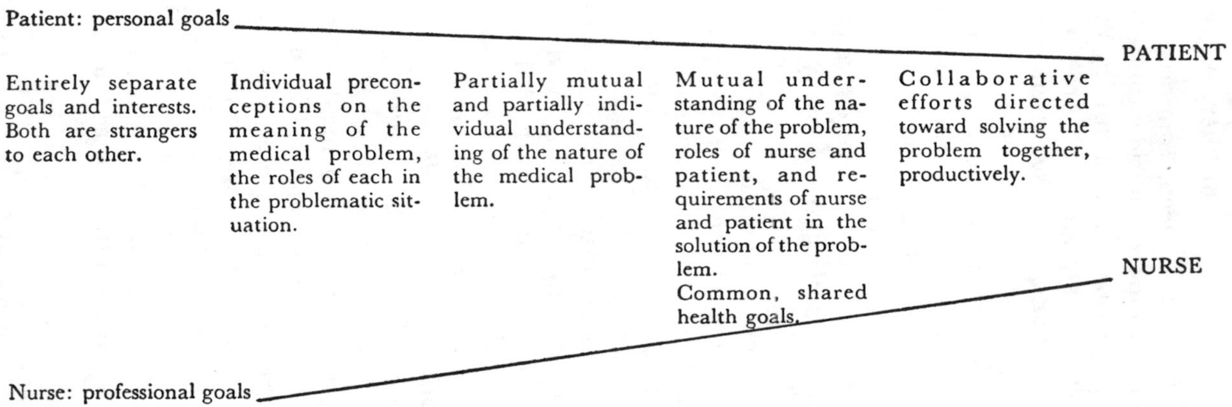

Patient: personal goals

PATIENT

Entirely separate goals and interests. Both are strangers to each other.

Individual preconceptions on the meaning of the medical problem, the roles of each in the problematic situation.

Partially mutual and partially individual understanding of the nature of the medical problem.

Mutual understanding of the nature of the problem, roles of nurse and patient, and requirements of nurse and patient in the solution of the problem.

Common, shared health goals.

Collaborative efforts directed toward solving the problem together, productively.

Nurse: professional goals

NURSE

Fig. 2. A continuum showing changing aspects of nurse-patient relations.

dividuals with separate goals and interests; at the other end are two persons working together to solve a presenting difficulty about which there are common understandings. (See Fig. 2, p. 10.) At any given time the relationship falls at a point on the continuum. The functions, roles, judgments in practice, and skills that demand scientific knowledge and technical abilities of many kinds change as the relationship of nurse to patient moves from point to point along the range of the continuum. Human contacts in nursing situations are extremely intimate ones.[4] Since human needs find expression in demands that may be overt or subtle and operate two ways in the nurse-patient situation, it is necessary that self-insight operate as an essential tool and as a check in all nurse-patient relationships that are meant to be therapeutic.

What can nursing do as a therapeutic, educative instrument and as a professional function of a health team? Health is the goal of all professional services. Do we know what the conditions are that promote "physical, emotional, and social well-being"? Do we know enough about what is meant by health to speculate on what conditions are required to promote it on the widest possible scale for all of the people? Do professional health teams that are developing rapidly within institutions and social agencies know how to organize their efforts so that public interest can be mobilized to support provision of conditions required for health? What part can nursing play in the interrelation of professional functions that gradually provide conditions suitable for health improvement? These are questions that concern nurses. They point to the urgent need for studying the nursing process in situations where it is effective and where it fails. They point to the immediacy of the need for nurses to know what tasks are being demanded of them in nursing situations. In this work we are particularly concerned with delineating the

[4] Helen Sargent, "Professional Ethics and Problems of Therapy," *The Journal of Abnormal and Social Psychology*, Vol. 40, No. 1 (January, 1945), p. 47. Makes a similar assertion with regard to client relationships with psychologists, psychiatrists, and social workers.

psychological tasks that develop in interpeisonal situations, particularly in the nurse-patient relationship. What nursing is and what it can become depend upon how well nurses can recognize the difficulties encountered in relations with people, and how skillful they become in helping people to resolve their difficulties and to develop new skills in meeting recurring problems.

Nurses do not have an exclusive or a prior claim on bringing about healthful living but share this objective with many other professional workers. They do have an area of operation that is unique, for example, in the care of sick people, and in which they carry a major responsibility. Nurses also share the responsibility for stating, in co-operation with other professional workers, criteria for desirable living and for working out policies and plans for achieving conditions that make health possible, Health has not been clearly defined; it is a word symbol that implies forward movement of personality and other ongoing human processes in the direction of creative, constructive, productive, personal, and community living.[5]

With this definition of health in mind, it can be seen that *nurses participate with other professional workers in the organization of conditions that facilitate forward movement of personality and other ongoing human processes in the direction of creative, constructive, productive, personal, and community living.* What are some of the human processes that lead in the direction of health? If nursing is to function co-operatively with them and to aid in organizing conditions that facilitate ongoing tendencies, there is need to identify what they are. One of the more obvious ones would include all of the biological ongoing processes: assimilation, absorption, elimination, etc. Nursing has always indentified itself as being on the side of preserving and conserving life, as

[5] For a statement of desirable characteristics of healthful living, see: Delbert Obertauffer, *Social Health Education* (New York, Harper & Brothers, 1949). Quoting from, The Faculty of Ohio State University, Department of University Schools, *A Report of the Health Committee* (Columbus, Ohio, 1942), p. 2, mimeographed.

opposed to movements that offer more rapid death to chronic sufferers and slowly dying patients. Pediatric nursing seeks to learn what are the biological developmental tasks required of growing infants and small children so that its functions can be geared to aid the ongoing processes of child development. Obstetric nursing is investigating Natural Childbirth, or Physiological Childbirth as it is referred to more recently, so that its techniques and functions can be improved in support of the natural human processes that operate during delivery of a pregnant woman. And, more importantly, so that the mother may share in accomplishing the delivery of her child.

There are other human processes that are of social origin. Education, medicine, social work, nursing, and a host of other professions and social institutions and agencies have their origins in human insights and desires to influence progress in meeting human needs. It is pretty well established that the mind develops in and through the social process or milieu into which the human organism is born, and that it is a process that represents total human functioning, in contrast to the functioning of a particular body organ—there being none from which the mind specifically draws its stimulation and right to function.

The hospital ward as a social context in which the patient can be aided to grow in the direction of health requires investigation into conditions it provides that facilitate promotion of "physical, emotional, and social well-being." Nurses have primary responsibility for development and improvement of this social context so that growth can take place. Human needs of patients are expressed within the limitations of this context and are responded to by professional persons directly connected with its development and improvement.

If nursing is to function in co-operation with internal and external human processes it will be necessary to have knowledge of particular processes and their relationship to the solution of specific interpersonal problems, such as: "Why won't John Jones eat?" In order to understand this problem fully and to arrive at mature judgment on how it best can be handled in co-operation with John Jones, it is necessary to know principles of biological and physical sciences, principles of social and psychological sciences, as they relate to to this individual problem. Nursing, as an applied science, develops its principles by interrelating ones from all other known sciences and applying them to everyday nursing problems. Knowing principles that govern or elucidate functioning of human processes, knowing conditions that are required for ameliorating dysfunctioning, and being able to develop experiences that apply such knowledge and lead in the direction of health are all required in nursing.

Conditions that will facilitate natural ongoing tendencies in any human organism are investigated by studying particular problems that arise in the life of a patient, his family, and his community. Each problem has unique factors to be considered. However, general conditions that are likely to lead to health always include the interpersonal environment, with which the remainder of this book is concerned. Other conditions include biological needs, such as tissue needs for fluids, for vitamins, endocrine substances, and the like. Physiological functioning often requires surgical removal of an organ, repair of an impediment, dietary manipulations, supportive medications; all require organization. The conditions that lead toward health cannot be presented in a haphazard way and then be used intelligently. Conditions that support processes of self-repair and self-renewal are psychobiological and can be separated only for purposes of clarifying aspects of discussion.

Two general categories summarize interacting conditions essential for experiencing health. They are:

1. Physiological demands of a human organism that require material conditions manipulated in behalf of the welfare of an individual or group.
2. Interpersonal conditions, that are individual and social,

and that meet personality needs and allow the expression and use of capacities in a productive way.

Conditions required for healthful physiological functioning cannot always be provided. They sometimes depend upon limited scientific knowledge. Often a problem comes to the attention of a health team after a need has been problematic too long. Enough has not yet been established as fact to arrest all pathological processes and to reverse physiological functioning in the direction of self-repair as, for example, in advanced carcinomatous growth and extensive tuberculous lesions. It is likewise true that psychoses of long duration are not readily reversed. Prevention in the area of physiological and of psychological functioning is largely a matter of identifying a situation that has become problematic early enough to be able to do something constructive about it by means that are available. Recent emphases on early detection of threats to health, such as cancer, tuberculosis, and the like, are indicated in the movement toward developing multiphasic health clinics as a part of health centers or outpatient departments. Recognizing limits to what the health service professions can now do, in relation to common health problems faced everyday, by no means negate the fact that *as conditions essential for health are more fully known and are provided and used by individuals and communities, more and more individuals will be enabled to experience greater health.*

What interpersonal conditions are required in order that health may be experienced? What is required in the nurse-patient relationship and in hospital wards as a social context in which growth can take place? How can competent nursing facilitate the forward movement of personality? How can nursing function as a maturing force in ordinary nursing situations? Are more nurses planning to leave the bedside or to cease visiting in homes of the sick in order to educate people? These are crucial questions being raised every day.

These are the issues that demand that nursing define what it can do in its unique spheres of operation. These are the problems that demand that each nurse examine the concept of nursing under which she operates.

Summary of nursing concept

Nursing is determined in situations in collaboration with other professional workers and occasionally at this time by what others permit a nurse to view as the functions of nursing. Nurses are available to patients in hospitals over a longer period of time than any worker in the health services. The round-the-clock demands of patients can only be heeded, currently, in terms of what is permitted by all workers in a particular situation. In some situations nursing can expand readily and thus fulfill its larger social obligation; in others, nursing is restricted to stereotyped functions. In each situation, the readiness of nurses to work for opportunity to think for themselves and to share in the determination of what can be done to meet patient needs, or their readiness to permit others to make all decisions and govern all of their actions, is an important factor in defining nursing and what it can do. For purposes of this book, the concept of nursing that is herewith accepted and that underlies the concepts presented is summarized as follows:

Nursing is a significant, therapeutic, interpersonal process. It functions co-operatively with other human processes that make health possible for individuals in communities. In specific situations in which a professional health team offers health services, nurses participate in the organization of conditions that facilitate natural ongoing tendencies in human organisms. Nursing is an educative instrument, a maturing force, that aims to promote forward movement of personality in the direction of creative, constructive, productive, personal, and community living.

CHAPTER 2

Phases of Nurse-patient Relationships

Overview

IN THIS CHAPTER four overlapping phases of nurse-patient relationships will be considered. In order to recognize and study what happens in a nurse-patient relationship, it is helpful to delineate aspects of the total situation. While there appear to be four clearly discernible phases in the relationship—orientation, identification, exploitation, and resolution—these are to be thought of as interlocking. (See Fig. 3, p. 21.) Each phase is characterized by overlapping roles or functions in relation to health problems as nurse and patient learn to work co-operatively to resolve difficulties. Each phase defines tasks and roles required of the nurse in the situation. These four units can be recognized; they enter into every total nursing situation.

Essential questions

How do different people react when they first feel ill? Do they always seek professional help? When they do seek professional help, what kinds of attitudes characterize their behavior? Do people generally know how to use professional help? How do they learn to seek and use help? Do you make people more dependent when you offer help? If you help people over a long period of time, do they always want to free themselves and become independent of it? What is a healthy attitude toward dependence and independence? How should an individual feel about being sick? How does an individual feel about getting nursing care from a stranger? Out of questions like these inquiry into the phases of a nurse-patient relationship can be developed.

Phase of orientation

Different individuals react differently to illness. In this inquiry we are interested in what happens when an ill person and a nurse come together to resolve a difficulty felt in relation to health. Many patients visit their private physicians and through them seek admission to hospitals for further study or treatment. Others may call upon a public health nursing agency for assistance. In each of these instances two basic factors stand out: (1) There is a "felt need"; a health problem has emerged and is more or less clear to the individual. (2) Professional assistance that is thought to be helpful is sought. These two factors indicate that the patient has an impression that he requires help in order to face a problem. He may need that assistance immediately, as in an emergency, or he may have opportunity to make plans for getting the help at some future date, as in scheduling ahead for an operation that is needed but is not imperative.

Seeking assistance on the basis of felt need is an important aspect of the phase of orientation. It makes a great deal of difference in the outcome for the patient, from the standpoint of personality expansion, how the nurse feels about helping others. What are some of the different ways that one can feel about giving help? Are there selective responses depending upon the extent of need that seems apparent? Does it make a difference if the patient arrives in the hospital at eleven in the morning, when most of the morning care is completed, or if he arrives when a nurse responsible for his admission is completing her work for the day? Does the age of the patient make a difference in how certain nurses feel? Does the kind of help that is required make it easier or more difficult to accept the patient as he is? How does the nurse feel about patients who come by stretcher and those who walk into a hospital?

Seeking assistance on the basis of a need, felt but poorly understood, is often the first step in a dynamic learning experience from which a constructive next step in personal-social growth can occur. Viewing illness as a learning experience will not change a nurse's feeling about giving help to people unless the school of nursing also permits and provides an appropriate setting, or social context, in which it is possible for student nurses to identify their feelings and to reorient them. However, patients do adapt to the situation or they learn something as an outcome of experiencing illness and nursing. Nurses are eager that the learning will be constructive. Modern curriculum experts are advocating that school teachers develop "real life experiences" for young students in order that meaningful learning will occur Nearly every minute of a nurse's day is involved in real life experiences that are new, problematic, and often dramatic. The opportunities for learning on the part of patients and nurses are many.

What practical difference does it make if nursing situations are viewed as learning experiences? Does it make a difference in how the primary goal is viewed? If the immediate conquering of disease is considered first and the primary problem viewed as destroying invading organisms, surgically removing obstructing structures, or removing symptoms of disordered personality functioning, is it more likely that all workers on the professional team will organize conditions with major emphasis on eradication and/or removal? If the relationship of the event itself to the personal-social growth of the individual is given primary emphasis—the experience viewed as an event that involves the possibility of learning— is there greater chance of organizing conditions for solving the problem to include genuine consideration of the personality needs of the individual who is ill? In which course of action are the feelings and attitudes of the patient more likely to be given full consideration from the outset?

It is conceivable that cures may be effected but that patients cannot be aided to experience health unless nursing situations are developed with full consideration of the educative needs of patients. The authority of the situation itself determines the necessity for immediacy of nursing action or possibilities for delay until the patient can be helped to understand and participate in prescribed treatment. *Nurses respond to situations in which emergencies carry authority that demand emergency responses:* the question of understanding, participation, consent does not enter into consideration of whether a patient shall be prevented from suicidal attempt or whether hemorrhage shall be stopped. Beyond the few life-or-death situations are many that fall under the well-known title of routine care, where the educative needs of the patient can be considered.

What kinds of educative needs might a patient have during a phase called orientation? What does the patient need to know about his present situation in order to resolve the difficulty and develop his personality further? How can a nurse help a patient become aware of what is happening to him in the present? We have already said that the patient has an impression about his problem. How can the nurse help the patient to expand this impression, so that the difficulty can be more fully understood and co-operative behavior established?

The patient often provides leads on how he visualizes the difficulty, providing opportunities for a nurse to recognize gaps in information and understanding. Frequently patients will ask questions: What is wrong with me? Why should this thing happen to me? What caused it? How will it turn out? What can the doctor do? These questions show how an individual attempts to expand an initial impression in order to get clear on the meaning of an experience that is being undergone. Nursing functions aid this process of clarification so that the experience can be integrated by the patient, as one in which meaningful learning has occurred.

During orientation as well as during the other three phases in the total relationship four interlocking nursing functions may operate:[1] (1) A nurse may function in the role of *resource person*, giving specific, needed information that aids the pa-

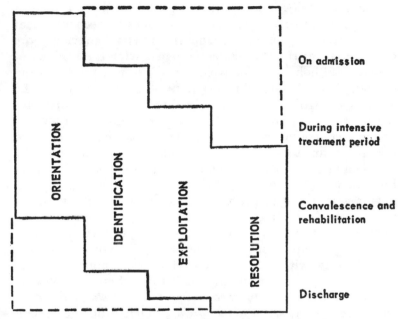

Fig. 3.   Overlapping phases in nurse-patient relationships.

tient to understand his problem and the new situation. (2) A nurse may function in a *counseling relationship*, listening to the patient as he reviews events that led up to his hospitalization and his feelings connected with them. (3) The patient may cast the nurse into roles, such as *surrogate* for mother, father, sibling, in which the nurse aids the patient by permitting him to re-enact and examine generically older feelings

[1] See Chapter 3 for full discussion.

generated in prior relationships. Effective performance in these roles provides the patient with a new symbol of authority or rivalry figures, and permits him to reorient his feelings relative to them. (4) The nurse also functions as a *technical expert,* who understands various professional devices and can manipulate them with skill and discrimination in the interest of the patient.

The patient does not usually recognize that these four functions can be available for his use nor does he recognize that his requirements often demand them. His behavior more often indicates that he has certain needs for these kinds of professional help. (1) The patient needs to recognize and understand his difficulty and the extent of need for help; (2) he needs to recognize and to be helped to plan to use what professional services can offer; (3) energy deriving from tension and anxiety connected with "felt needs" can be harnessed to positive means for defining, understanding, and meeting the problem at hand. Each patient seeks these kinds of help in his own way. Interpreting these tasks from the patient's behavior is required of professional workers and the patient's perceptions of their responses constitute an orientation for him, toward the new, presenting, learning experience in the situation in which he now finds himself. Nurses function participantly with all members of a professional team as they aid the patient in making orienting differentiations.

The patient needs to recognize and understand his difficulty and the extent of need for help. Orienting the patient to what is involved in his problem is a complex task. In some situations it will be possible for nurses to function as resource persons, conveying specific information and assisting the patient to see relations to symptoms that accompany his illness. Thus, a patient whose difficulty is diagnosed as diabetes can be aided to understand relationships between his symptoms, laboratory findings, and dietary procedures. His future behavior can be determined by him, in light of knowledge the nurse shares with him. This function is not permitted in all situations or in relation to all disease categories; these matters need to be worked out with professional personnel in specific situations.

Recognizing the full import of the nuclear problem and the kind of professional assistance that is needed is largely the task of evaluating and diagnosing the emergent problem. This function is primarily that of a physician, functioning co-operatively with technical experts and in consideration of their reports and findings. Nursing functions assist in gathering observable objective data, in reinforcing and clarifying what the physician has communicated to the patient, and in identifying peripheral or sub-problems related to the main one.

To encourage the patient to participate in identifying and assessing his problem is to engage him as an active partner in an enterprise of great concern to him. Democratic method applied to nursing requires patient participation. It depends upon working toward consent and understanding of prevailing problems, related reality factors, and existing conditions by all participants. The power for accomplishing the tasks at hand, in ways that develop or expand personality, resides in the consent and understanding that motivate all persons concerned. By this definition of democratic power, many patients, or community members affected by an emergent difficulty, are powerless. Community health education consists in providing the public with sources of facts, on which its judgments, actions, and new values can be based. The principle is identical in hospital and home situations where the nurse-patient situation provides a more intimate setting for a tutorial kind of teaching. The patient, when aided in identifying and understanding facets of his medical problem, so he recognizes what is involved, can base his consent and subsequent actions on known data. A hospital incident exemplifies nurse participation in this needed orientation:

A professional nurse attending to the needs of a child recently admitted to a hospital who spoke and understood only Greek language, observed that the child was apprehensive in the new situation. She knew that the child did not understand what was happening to her. When an intern entered the room, stating, "Get her ready for an intravenous," the nurse replied, "We are not ready yet. I wish to speak to you outside." When the intern insisted that he had everything that was needed on the intravenous tray, the nurse merely repeated her first reply in calm, but firm, manner. Outside the room she related that the child was apprehensive and that it would be necessary for her to prepare the child psychologically for the intravenous procedure before the intern could proceed in carrying it out. When the intern returned later the procedure was carried out with full consent and interest on the part of the patient.

This example of need for orientation to an aspect of hospital experience is in contrast to ones many nurses have observed or felt obliged to participate in. Another example is children taken to the operating room before full consent and orientation to the situation has been achieved. Many a patient perfectly able to understand and to share in some of the facts about *his* medical problem is denied opportunity for participating in this important event in *his* life. Yet such *orientation is essential to full participation and to full integration of the illness event into the stream of life experiences* of the patient. *It is the only prevention against repressing or dissociating the event that a nurse can exercise* on behalf of the patient. The patient's problem becomes more complex when there is need to ignore or deny aspects of the present situation in order to feel comfortable in it, as indicated in the following illustration of dissociation of a wish that previously had been in awareness of the patient. A young girl was admitted to a hospital for an exploratory abdominal operation; it was expected that the surgeon would need to remove one ovary and the patient was told that this would be the extent of the operative intervention. She casually mentioned to one of the nurses that she was hoping to get married soon and that she and her boy friend were planning to have a family. However, the nurse commented, "Isn't that wonderful," making no reference to its possible relationship to the impending operation. Following the operation and recovery from anesthesia, the patient was told, rather summarily, that it had been found necessary to remove her uterus and both ovaries. The nurses noted that there were marked changes in the patient's personality thereafter; she was quiet, passive, uncomplaining, and never discussed her future plans nor did she show interest in being visited by her fiancé. These characteristics were in marked contrast to her enthusiasm and spontaneity on admission. It is conceivable that her wish to become a creative, productive woman and her feelings about the surgical destruction of her biological ability to move in this direction were dissociated. Nurses can speculate that assistance in orienting this patient to her difficulty and her feelings connected with possible outcomes might have been more useful prior to operation and that subsequent effects may now require intensive psychotherapeutic assistance at some future date. They can also speculate that the nurse's comment, "Isn't that wonderful," closed off the possibility of further clarification of what the patient was actually feeling at that time.

The patient needs assistance in recognizing and planning to use services that professional personnel can offer. Meeting this task is a joint responsibility of medical and nursing staff and requires co-operative planning. Unless there is agreement among all workers who come into contact with the patient on what is a desirable course of action in relation to his problem, their disagreement may communicate itself to the patient whose discomfort may then interfere with achievement of treatment goals.[2] When treatment plans are developed through collaboration, concerted interest in the patient can more easily be demonstrated.

Nursing is particularly concerned in orienting and informing the patient of provisions and limits that affect available hospital service. These provisions have to do with nursing

[2] Alfred H. Stanton and Morris S. Schwartz, "The Management of a Type of Institutional Participation in Mental Illness," *Psychiatry*, Vol. XII, No. 1 (February, 1949), p. 18. An important paper that shows that disagreements between nurses that cannot be openly discussed are acted out in nursing situations and distort the nurse-patient relationship.

services: the bedside nurse will be available to the patient during certain periods—for the bath, following anesthesia, while carrying out procedures, for distribution of medicines. Moreover, the call bell is available for bringing nurse to patient, for attending to other needs as they arise. Situational limits, such as visiting hours, care of flowers, cleaning of the room, mail delivery, when pointed out as the patient is orienting himself to this new psychological situation makes it possible for him to begin to organize his activities in terms of what is permitted. Knowledge of hospital services to be placed at the disposal of the patient helps him to feel secure that something will be done to meet and satisfy his needs and wants. Limitations represent cultural boundaries—standards or rules of conduct that constitute the hospital's administrative expectations of the patient. When these expectations are made clear in the beginning, the patient can visualize boundaries and use his energies to harmonize his needs and goals with them. He can more readily feel certain that the hospital experience will prove to be an orderly and helpful one to him.

Every institution and agency can ask itself: What can we offer patients and how can we inform them during an initial orientation period, in a way that is clarifying rather than confusing? Methods may differ but the principle remains the same; when a patient is left in doubt about ordinary services that are available for his use he becomes more anxious and uncertain about the wisdom of the present course of action.

Every patient needs to be assisted in harnessing energy that derives from tension and anxiety connected with felt needs, to positive means for defining, understanding, and meeting productively the problem at hand. The patient admitted to a hospital is likely to be overawed by the activity surrounding his admission. If anxiety is felt at all it is likely to be overlooked by the nurse in the welter of details connected with the patient's orientation. Nevertheless, unless real consideration is given to this most important aspect in the orientation period, the tone for all later relationships in the hospital experience may be set at a level below that needed for integrating the present event into the stream of life experiences.

What aspects of personality are threatened by admission to a hospital? Why does a patient develop tension and anxiety during a clinic visit? Why do patients appear upset and uncomfortable when a nurse visits their home? Tension or anxiety is usually present in some degree and may or may not be observable. Depending upon the patient's characteristic pattern of responding in crisic situations, anxiety may develop rapidly in relation to threats of separation from family members. Particularly when the patient is separated from someone on whom he has been most dependent, such as wife or mother. If relatives are rudely or abruptly separated from the patient, so that he feels cut off from supportive and sustaining relationships, before similar ones seem likely in the new situation, older responses to prior experiences may be reactivated. Severe anxiety may develop. Apathy, dependence, or overaggression may characterize the behavioral response. Alertness to those situations where anxiety may convert into terror or panic requires flexibility in executing hospital administrative policies, so that they will not operate to the disfavor of the patient.

If for reasons of expediency the nurse must ask relatives to leave immediately, ample warning and clear explanation of what is to be done permit the patient to anticipate a new event and to receive reassurance from familiar persons. Everything that is done with the patient or within his hearing requires an orienting explanation. All personnel can introduce themselves or be introduced when they ordinarily come in contact with the patient, as natural functions are carried out. Every request or anticipated need of the newly admitted patient when met with interest and a genuine wish to serve the purpose of the hospitalization experience help the patient to feel that he is accepted in the new situation.

The very fact of illness and confinement to a room or ward constricts the life space of the patient and focusses his attention on smaller and smaller details. A busy nurse who has many important larger problems to handle or unimportant busywork to focus upon may easily take it for granted that the patient either understands what is going on about him or that he has not perceived anything of importance. The patient is then left to develop the meaning of everyday events without recourse to previous experiences that were similar. *The limitations in life space and on freedom of movement thrust the patient back on his own imagination, or upon the guidance of hospital personnel, for clarification and explanation of what is happening around him.* When a professional nurse arranges time for aiding the patient in becoming oriented to the mores and customs of the hospital or agency and to seeing relations of its services to his problem, the experience in the hospital is likely to be characterized by useful learning.

Clarifying with the patient aspects of the situation, procedures to be carried out, events that occur around him provide contacts for observing and finding out what the patient expects of nurses and how he feels about illness. Expectations and feelings are also expressed in responses the patient selectively makes to concrete experiences with nursing care. Different patients have different expectations of nursing; most patients have mixed feelings about their illness. Many patients cannot state what they feel. "I feel uncomfortable," "I don't feel good," "I am miserable" are common ways of expressing the dilemma that feelings are mixed and poorly understood. The nurse who responds unconditionally, that is, making no demands upon the patient to satisfy her own needs rather than his own, orienting the patient toward focusing on the problem, will permit the patient to express *his* feelings so that he can become aware of what they are. Advice, reassurance, suggestion, persuasion are of little value when offered in connection with feelings. For example, a patient admitted to the hospital remarks to the nurse, "I certainly wish I could go home. I don't want to stay here." When a nurse responds by saying, "Oh, we will take good care of you," the patient may feel ashamed to reveal himself further. When a nurse says, "You don't want to stay, you would feel more comfortable at home," the patient is not deflected from focusing on the feelings that underlie his remark. If he senses that the nurse is a friendly person, and if he is an individual who can confide in others, he may expand his first remark. He may say, "Yes, I think of hospitals as places to go to when you are dying and I don't want to die." Again, a nurse may believe the way to reassure the patient is by showing him that his feelings are not to be trusted, she may say, "Oh, but you aren't going to die, we will take care of you." This remark, in effect, denies the validity of the patient's feelings and in order to feel safe the patient may have to give up attending to what he feels and indicate verbal acceptance of what the nurse has indicated he *should* feel. In contrast, a nurse might respond by saying, "You want to live and you feel afraid that you might not if you stay here." This open comment permits the patient to examine his feelings still further if he wishes and thus it provides an opportunity for him to orient himself in this new situation in terms of what he actually feels. Awareness of feelings develops understanding of the situation as it is seen by the patient and thus leads to the possibility of voluntary control and appropriate nurse actions.

Nondirective listening offers the patient a sounding board against which he can reveal feelings and discover them. The patient feels what *he* feels; he cannot reorient his feelings to what others expect of him until he is aware of them. The presence of an intelligent listener is of value; suggestions are intrusions that are likely to disorient the patient in the task at hand—finding out what he feels about his present state of affairs.

Initially, the patient functions in relation to overlapping situations. That is, he is pulled toward being home where he is sure of familiar responses and he is drawn toward remaining in the hospital and solving the emergent problem. As the home and hospital situations merge into one concept that pulls together, taking the patient in the direction of a solution to his difficulty, the patient can become better able to focalize on the tasks to be accomplished. This outcome cannot occur at once but takes time and demonstrated interest on the part of hospital personnel. It requires co-operation with the family. It requires that the patient become sufficiently oriented to the hospital situation so that needs ordinarily met in the family can find outlet in the new situation. Needs for care, comfort, shared goals, sustaining relationships, feelings of acceptance—these are all shared temporarily with the family, as nurse and patient focus on a presenting medical problem.

During the period of orientation the patient clarifies his first, whole impression of his problem; facets of it are expanded and details connected with it become clear as the people in the new psychological situation act in relation to the patient. The patient participates in the orienting process by asking questions, by trying to find out what he needs to know in order to feel secure, and by observing ways in which professional people respond with him. By asking for help, in receiving assistance, the patient soon begins to feel at home, so to speak, knowing that his wants will be permitted expression and taken care of.

Phase of identification

When the patient's first impression is somewhat clarified, and he feels that he knows what the situation can offer him, he responds selectively to persons who seem to offer the help that he needs. This phase may be called identification.

Some patients will feel as if they belong and are part of this venture of dealing with a problem connected with illness. They take on the attitudes of cheerfulness, optimism, and problem-solving as they identify with nurses who are themselves cheerful, optimistic, and helpful in the solution of problems. These patients will feel stronger and less powerless in the face of illness; often there is a feeling that "things are going to be all right."

These patients may explore many feelings that the culture does not ordinarily approve—feelings of helplessness, dependency, self-centeredness, the wish to cry, and the like. Patients reveal these feelings when they feel safe in professional hands. *When a nurse permits patients to express what they feel, and still get all of the nursing that is needed, then patients can undergo illness as an experience that reorients feelings and strengthens positive forces in personality.* Feelings of helplessness, or crying, are sometimes viewed as behavior that is "put on" for the benefit of nurse or family in order to get attention. If sustained assistance or self-enhancement are not provided in other ways patients often do use, unwittingly, these forms of behavior to express the powerlessness that they feel. Ordinarily, illness is felt as a threat to security, to power, to feelings of dignity and worthwhileness. These feelings are minimized as the patient identifies with persons who help him to feel less threatened. Nursing symbolizes acceptance of people as they are and assistance in times of stress.

Not every patient can easily identify and ally himself with others who accept him. Often earlier interpersonal relationships have been so traumatic that it seems inconceivable to the patient that others can accept him as he is. Some patients feel that they must not make demands upon nursing; these patients tend to isolate themselves and are inclined to want to be independent of any kind of help. The meaning of the symbol nursing cannot be absorbed because the patient is unable to refer to an earlier experience where the meaning operated in a human relationship.[3] Nursing can develop and offer experiences that are new and rewarding and enable the patient to identify sufficiently for expression of feelings. Nursing needs to inquire into the possibilities of using nurse-patient relationships, and its natural vehicles in nursing care, such as the bath, feeding, giving enemas, as new experiences in "mothering" that displace earlier traumatic childhood

[3] Nathaniel Cantor, *Dynamics of Learning* (Buffalo, New York, Foster and Stewart Publishing Corporation, 1946), p. 26.

experiences. Developing the feeling of being related to others in a way that allows expression of underlying needs and wishes is possible in nursing situations.

Some patients identify too readily with nurses, expecting that all of their wants will be taken care of and nothing will be expected of them. These patients may go through the phase of orientation very quickly, being little concerned about participating in the process of attacking problems and formulating solutions. Everything is left in the hands of others who will take care of them. The pattern of overdependence on forces outside of the self for solution of common, everyday problems is a crucial social issue. At the present level of cultural achievement there are large numbers of people who cannot seem to meet crises constructively.[4, 5] One individual in every ten will at some time during his life require hospitalization for psychiatric treatment; large numbers of general hospital patients show emotional difficulties in addition to organic dysfunctioning; large numbers of individuals assuage their feelings of helplessness by resorting to drugs, alcohol, or other pseudosolutions to their problems; suicide, delinquency, murder, all of these forms of participation in life indicate the extent of helplessness among the general population to cope with individual crises in ways that are constructive and promote growth.

Nursing needs to ask itself this question; can the nurse-patient relationship be developed so that it facilitates forward movement of personality in ways that displace feelings of helplessness and powerlessness with feelings of creativeness, spontaneity, and productivity? Can these products be fostered in a fruitful nurse-patient relationship? How can nursing provide direct experiences with helpful persons that diminish feelings of helplessness in patients? All nursing situations

[4] See statement of Brock Chisolm (M.D.), *Proceedings of the National Conference of Social Work,* published for the National Conference of Social Work (New York, Columbia University Press, 1947), pp. 48-49.

[5] For further identification of this problem see George S. Stevenson (M.D.), "Yardstick for Citizenship," *The Survey,* Vol. LXXXV, No. 7 (July, 1949), p. 357.

take place under the urgency of need, in some degree. Can they be developed so that the experience will move in the direction of a more mature person-to-person relationship, in which neither nurse or patient feels helpless?

During the period of identification, when quality nursing is provided, the patient may be renourished by these events that psychologically take him back to childhood ways.[6] Three ways in which patients respond during this phase have been identified: (1) on the basis of participation or interdependent relations with a nurse; (2) on the basis of independence or isolation from a nurse; (3) on the basis of helplessness or dependence upon a nurse. The phases of orientation and identification are essentially like those stages of passive-receptivity and identification noted during infancy or the early oral stage of personality development.[7] Psychologically, the patient experiences degrees of the same feelings that operated at any earlier stage in his life. There is the complicating factor of chronological age and the imposition of cultural factors on the patient's view of himself. It may not be a simple achievement for the patient to permit expression of babylike feelings. It is as if the patient wishes to reassure himself that he has control beyond the extent indicated in his feelings. Quality nursing is perceptive of both the psychological feelings and the cultural counterfeelings and attempts to help the patient to experience both with a minimum of interference to the outcome of his illness. Most patients, after they have explored their wishes to maintain their usual adult behavior in doing things for themselves during a serious illness, arrive at full recognition of their need for help and can accept it. Nurses can point out the temporary nature of the need for complete, dependent care—when this is vital to the treatment goal—and help the patient to keep the wish to be an adult alive. As conditions permit most patients can be helped to help themselves in the nursing care process. A

[6] See, for example: Samuel Z. Orgel, "Identification as a Socializing and Therapeutic Force," *American Journal Orthopsychiatry*, 11:118 (1941).
[7] See Chapter 4.

Basic Principles in learning theory*	Leadership functions during phase of Identification		Leadership functions during phase of Resolution	
	Behavior of nurse in leadership role.	Behavior of patient as follower.	Behavior of nurse in leadership role.	Behavior of patient as follower.
Drive	For recognition and approbation of the physician.	For recognition and approbation of the physician.	For recognition and approbation of the physician.	For recognition and approbation of the physician.
Cue	Plan of treatment outlined, re taking fluids.	Fluids offered by the nurse.	Plan of treatment outlined, re taking fluids.	Understanding of plan of treatment and goals.
Response	Provides fluids and sees that patient drinks.	Takes fluids (*i.e.*, responds to cue from nurse).	Provides fluids when patient requests (*i.e.*, responds to cues from patient).	Asks for fluids and keeps own record of intake.
Reward	Recognition and approbation from physician for responding to cue in nursing plan.	Recognition and approbation from physician for responding to cue from nurse.	Recognition and approbation from physician for engendering sound learning in patient.	Recognition and approbation from physician for responding to own cues perceived as participant.
Learning	To respond to own cues and get reward.	To respond to cues from nurse to get reward.	To foster learning in patients is rewarding.	To respond to crucial cues in situation and get reward for own efforts.

* References: J. Dollard and N. E. Miller, *Social Learning and Imitation.* New Haven, Conn., Yale University Press, 1941.

Fig. 4. Role of leadership functions in two phases in a nurse-patient relationship, involving fluid intake.

number of significant papers in Witmer, *Teaching Psychotherapeutic Medicine*, elaborate this point.[8]

It is important that nurses keep in mind the leadership role into which the patient casts her and its relations to identification. Identification makes possible imitative learning, but this is not the goal in the learning experience being developed with the patient. Constructive learning takes place when the patient can perceive and focus on crucial cues in the situation, through his own efforts, and when he can develop responses to them independently of the nurse.[9] This movement in perception and response is indicated in Fig. 4, p. 34.

Symonds points out that identification gives rise to mixed feelings of love and hatred.[10] Help is perceived as useful but the person who has power to help another may be envied or hated for the very skills that are respected. Expressing mixed feelings, in a situation where it is permitted, is advantageous, as Kauffman suggests.[11] Feelings of strength, assurance, personal power generate as the patient develops skills that involve personal effort. There is a difference felt by the patient who is required to let a *nurse do things for him, to do things for himself,* or *to work interdependently with a nurse* in accomplishing the tasks required by the problem. The development of a person to person relationship may include all three modes of accomplishing the work required for goal achievement. A relationship may start with one pattern of patient behavior and move through the other two, as a co-operative relationship develops.

Patients identify with nurses on the basis of services that are recognized as useful. They also identify with nurses on

[8] Helen Witmer, ed., *Teaching Psychotherapeutic Medicine* (New York, Commonwealth Fund, 1947). See papers by Dr. John M. Murray, pp. 89-90; by Dr. John Romano, p. 228; by Dr. Murray, p. 277; by Dr. Murray and Dr. Henry Brosin, p. 278.

[9] See also a film by S. R. Slavson, *Activity Group Therapy*, produced through the Jewish Board of Guardians, Columbia University, New York City.

[10] Percival Symonds, *The Dynamics of Human Adjustment* (New York, Appleton-Century-Crofts, Inc., 1946), p. 320.

[11] Witmer, *op. cit.*, p. 68.

the basis of earlier experiences; it is as if, below the level of awareness, a connection between the behavior of the nurse and the present feelings of the patient is perceived. When the nurse is viewed as a figure, symbolic of past experience, values and feelings held in relation to the older experience are reactivated and enter into the patient's expectations of the nurse. The behavior of the nurse—her appearance, mode of action, body gesture, manner of speaking—will be evaluated in terms of the patient's past experience. When that past experience has included feelings of hostility and interferences with the expression of wishes and desires, the patient may include these in his preconceptions and expectations of the nurse.

For example, a forty-year-old patient who has maintained strong ties with a mother may expect many of her qualities to be evident in the nurse. If his mother was tall, gray-haired, and dominating and if this patient gets along with a nurse who is tall, gray-haired, and dominating, it is likely that these similarities provide the basis for the patient's ready acceptance of the nurse. On the other hand, a young, warm, spontaneous nurse may have great difficulty in gaining acceptance from this patient. His preconceptions and expectations of women in authority are jeopardized by the young nurse's appearance and her attitudes and this makes him feel anxious. He cannot use his customary patterns of behavior as readily in the presence of a figure who represents a different kind of authority. Yet, greater learning is possible in the latter situation, which does not continue to reinforce fixed responses but allows for growth. However, the responsibility for developing the experience in a way that fosters learning, and in a way that does not allow the patient's anxiety to overwhelm him, belongs to the nurse, in this case, the young nurse.

Since a nurse cannot possibly know what is in the mind of a patient until there is some communication between them, it is necessary for her to be straightforward and inquiring about needs connected with the emergent problem. However, once the patient is oriented to the outer structure of the hospital situation, the nurse can bend her efforts toward finding out what the patient's preconceptions are about nurses. Observation during the period of identification has two main purposes: (1) the development of clarity about the patient's preconceptions and expectations of nurses and nursing;[12] (2) the development of clarity regarding the nurse's preconceptions and expectations of a particular patient and his skills in handling his problem. The patient learns how to make use of the nurse-patient relationship as both come to know and to respect one another, as persons who have likes and differences in opinions, in ways of looking at a situation, in responding to events. The nurse makes use of professional education and skill in aiding the patient to arrive at a point where full use can be made of the relationship, in order to solve the medical problem. Further personality development occurs as a by-product of effective nursing.

Phase of exploitation

When a patient has identified with a nurse who can recognize and understand the interpersonal relations in the situation, the patient proceeds through a phase where he makes full use of the services offered to him. In various ways he attempts to derive full value from the relationship, in accordance with his view of the situation. All of the various goods and services at his disposal, as he has come to know them, will be exploited on the basis of self-interest and need.

If the patient feels fully at home, as if he belongs and is a participating member of the hospital family, and if he has a feeling of being comfortable and well taken care of, he will explore all of the possibilities of the changing situation. It sometimes can be observed that patients who are recuperating make more demands upon nursing than when their illness is more serious. Others patients are more self-directing and realistic about their exploitation of services. Actually,

---

[12] See Chapter 3 for full discussion of roles.

exploitative behavior is to be expected in some degree—the patient making full use of the nursing service offered—as though he were finding out and making sure that it is offered to him. Yet, at the same time, he begins to identify and to orient himself toward still other new goals, such as going home, returning to work, and the like.

The phase of exploitation overlaps identification and resolution, the terminal phase of the nurse-patient relationship. Orientation overlapped the previous social or home situation. The phase under discussion represents all prior ones and an extension of the self of the patient into the future. It is characterized by an intermingling of needs and a shuttling back and forth. Rapid shifts in behavior that express mixed needs makes observation more complex.

Behavior prior to and during convalescence, which begins during the exploitative phase, is more like the behavior of an adolescent.[13] The main difficulty seems to be that of trying to strike a balance between a need to be dependent, as during serious illness, and a need to be independent, as following recovery. Many patients experience these opposite feelings as conflict, vacillating between them and being unable to decide the direction in which they wish to move. The patient is served well when needs are met as they emerge, rather than calling specific attention to apparent inconsistencies perceived in behavior. Nursing has the task of understanding what gives rise to shifts in behavior.

There is always the possibility of the patient having exploitative character traits, and certainly these patients increase the complexity of the interpersonal situation. Within the limits of time of most hospital experiences it is impossible, indeed inadvisable, for a nurse to attempt to set up experiences or even to make any serious attempt to get at expression of such character traits. When manifested the problem is referable to the total function of the professional

[13] Witmer, *op. cit.*, p. 228. See also A. P. Solomon, "Rehabilitation of Patients with Psychologically Protracted Convalescence," *Archives of Physical Therapy*, 24:270-276 (1943).

team, for its decisions on approach to the difficulty. It is conceivable that in some patients, reinforcement of repressions may be indicated, unless personnel are prepared to handle the severe anxiety that might arise with admission into awareness of feelings connected with exploitative character needs. When these patients suffer a long-term illness, such as tuberculosis which requires prolonged hospital stay, they provide opportunities for exploring many possibilities in re-experiencing earlier events connected with anal functions, toilet training, and the learning of interference and delay in fulfilling personal wishes. The most complex nursing problems result from exploitation of the situation, not on the basis of positive identification with nurses and freedom for making use of services provided, but through an insatiable need to overpower, to dominate, to "get more than others" of what is available. Most mature nurses will find these patients challenging to their psychotherapeutic efforts.

Phase of resolution

As old needs are fully met they are gradually put aside willingly, by the patient himself, and aspirations are adapted to the new goals that were formulating while the patient was exploring and exploiting the use of nursing service. In relation to hospital practice it becomes discernible that the patient enters a stage of resolution. Old ties and dependencies are soon fully relinquished as the patient prepares to go home. If the home, through adequate educational preparation by public health nurses and social workers when this is possible, receives the patient in helpful ways and reinforces the therapeutic outcomes of the hospital experience, the illness event is soon integrated by the patient. The patient feels refreshed that in his time of troubles and helplessness, aid was actually forthcoming; this is a great fear of many people—that they may at some time be helpless and others will not care.

Logically, the stage of resolution should occur when the

medical or surgical problem is solved, the fever gone, the invading organism killed off, or the sutures removed and the incision fully healed and physical strength regained. However, since resolution is more a psychological phenomenon, medical recovery and the actual wish to terminate the event do not always coincide.[14] Nurses know of many patients who return to the hospital many times following discharge although no physical basis can be found to account for their recurring symptoms. Patients required to get out of bed under prescription of early ambulation are often eager and interested in their progress for the first few days, and then they begin to offer many complaints, which would seem to indicate that their dependency needs were not met earlier in the course of illness. It is not suggested that early ambulation is contraindicated; it is, however, pointed out that, when the patient is pushed physically, other ways must be found to make sure that felt needs for psychological dependency and for sustaining relationships are provided and worked through although the patient is able physically to take care of himself. When this principle is not recognized anxiety connected with unmet needs may be converted into vague symptoms that delay progress and at the same time utilize the tension in piecemeal fashion.

The stage of resolution implies the gradual freeing from identification with helping persons and the generation and strengthening of ability to stand more or less alone. These outcomes can be achieved only when all of the earlier phases are met in terms of *"psychological mothering": unconditional acceptance in a sustaining relationship that provides fully for need-satisfaction; recognition of and responses to growth cues, however trivial, as and when they come from the patient; shifting of power from the nurse to the patient as he*

[14] Virginia M. Axeline and Carl R. Rogers, "A Teacher-Therapist Deals with a Handicapped Child," *The Journal of Abnormal and Special Psychology*, Vol. 40, No. 2 (April, 1945), pp. 119-142. Case history of a child who failed to resolve his dependency needs in the hospital situation.

becomes willing to delay gratification of his wishes and to expend his own efforts in achieving new goals.[15]

Resolution is basically a freeing process; nursing helps the patient to organize his actions in this perspective during the entire hospital stay in order that it will be possible for the patient to want to be free for more productive social activities and relationships of his own choosing. What courses of action are required by nurses who wish patients to free themselves from dependency on others when crises have been met? Can a patient free himself if a nurse fixes all courses of action and evaluates attainment in these terms? Can a patient learn to free himself if his every move has been managed by someone else? Resolution is a freeing process but it depends for its possible success on the preceding chain of events.

Summary

When the serial and goal-directed nature of the nursing process is appreciated, nursing plans can be designed to include the steps necessary to make illness an eventful experience in learning for patients. Understanding of the meaning of the experience to the patient is required in order for nursing to function as an educative, therapeutic, maturing force. The patient's initial impression of a difficulty requires differentiation and expansion of all of the factors in the problem, as they affect him and his goals. Orientation to the problem leads to expression of needs and feelings, older ones that are reactivated and new ones created by challenges in a new situation. Identification with a nurse who consistently symbolizes a helping person, providing abundant and unconditional care, is a way of meeting felt needs and overwhelming problems. When initial needs are met they are outgrown and more mature needs arise. Exploiting what a situation offers gives rise to new differentiations

[15] For a related biological concept see Robert Briffault, *The Mothers* (New York, The Macmillan Company, 1937), Vol. I, p. 86.

of the problem and to the development and improvement of skill in interpersonal relations. New goals to be achieved through personal efforts can be projected. Movement from a hospital situation to participation in community life requires resolution of nurse-patient relations and the strengthening of personality for new social interdependent relationships. When resolution occurs on the basis of lacks in a situation needs are intensified and become longings that, together with unclear meanings of the event itself, limit the possibility of integration of the total experience. The nursing process can be systematically studied in nursing situations to test the validity of these hypotheses; a number of such studies are currently under way.

CHAPTER **3**

Roles in Nursing

Overview

MANY ROLES are demanded of nurses. Patients cast nurses into roles that seem necessary for meeting a problem as they view it. Nurses define roles in which they wish to function or that are thought to be desirable performances for a nurse. Society has views on how nurses should function and these conceptions vary in communities and economic groupings. Professional literature promotes pictures that influence nursing; textbooks on professional adjustments traditionally suggest patterns of behavior that indicate nursing roles. The purpose of this chapter is to examine some of the roles that emerge as the nursing process is studied in nurse-patient situations. It suggests principles that govern effective performance in the roles indicated.

Essential questions

What roles should a nurse fulfill? Are functions determined in advance or do they arise out of the authority of a situation? How does a patient view a nurse? Does the patient cast the nurse into roles that have a rational or a nonrational basis? Should a nurse respond in a nonrational role? Can a nurse shift her behavior from one role to another? Who should decide what roles a nurse can function in effectively? Should the physician decide? The patient? Society? All nurses? Each nurse? What practical difference does it make who decides? What is best for the patient? These are the important questions that nurses can discuss in order to illuminate the problem: What roles should a nurse fulfill? Understanding of the factors in these vital questions will provide a basis for designing nursing that is valuable to individuals and to society.

Role of stranger

It may surprise many nurses to realize that they are first a stranger to the patient. The patient is also a stranger to the nurse. This assertion poses the question: What expectations will a patient have on how this stranger, a nurse, will treat him? What kinds of performances has he a right to expect? How does the nurse feel about different strangers who arrive at the hospital under different circumstances? If the patient is not seen as a stranger, what stereotype of patient is operating in the nurse? Examination of these questions provides a framework for discussion of principles.

A stranger is an individual with whom another individual is not acquainted. When two strangers meet they have nothing in common of which they are aware. It doesn't matter whether the stranger arrives in the nurse's own home or in the hospital, the principle is the same: *respect and positive interest accorded a stranger is at first nonpersonal and includes the same ordinary courtesies that are accorded to a new guest who has been brought into any situation.* This principle implies: (1) accepting the patient as he is; (2) treating the patient as an emotionally able stranger and relating to him on this basis until evidence shows him to be otherwise.

Greeting a stranger cannot be stereotyped and sound genuine. An appropriate approach arises out of the personality of the nurse and the way she sizes up the situation. From the standpoint of patient expectations, it is useful to keep in mind that some aspects of the cultural view of a nurse are likely to operate and color what the patient expects will happen.[1]

Society has come to look upon nursing as a helping relationship on two accounts: (1) Nurses have portrayed themselves in this way in crises and thus established a favorable position of cultural prestige through their own efforts. (2) Since nursing is allied with the entire medical profession, society tends to view the physician as a person who understands and interprets the nature of the patient's problem while the nurse merely responds to and carries out his recommendations. In other words, the culture has rewarded nursing in terms of prestige for the ability of nurses to express a womanly role in an active way; it also takes cognizance of the passive aspect in total nursing functions. The valuable role played by male nurses is recognized; but, the culture usually refers to women when the symbol nurse comes to mind. Men and women nurses alike have very active roles to play in relation to the physician. Nurses must be able to interpret what is happening in the absence of the physician; often such interpretations have led to acts that have been life-saving for the patient. It is to be expected that the culture will cling to the stereotype of "nurse as handmaiden to the physician," and that responsibility for promoting a new view of the *nurse as associate with other professional workers* is a task of nursing.

The patient may develop expectations on the basis of the older concept of nursing. Many patients greet the nurse on arrival with such remarks as "Did my doctor tell you what to do for me, yet?" "Are you sure that this is what my doctor wants you to do?" How do nurses feel about strangers who so quickly and blithely threaten their need to feel that they are adequate to the circumstances of the patient's problem? Even though the nurse knows that in most hospitals she

[1] R. L. Birdwhistle, "Social Science and Nursing Education: some tentative suggestions," NLNE 1949 Fifty-ninth Annual Report, pp. 315-28.

cannot make a retort that could be considered "unprofessional," are there trigger responses in feelings that occur and that she feels must be vented elsewhere?

In some situations nurses harassed by an overwhelming burden of work may, on occasion, make a most inappropriate remark that distorts interpersonal relations. For example, a patient, multipara, admitted to a hospital at the height of a period of hectic activity was greeted by the remark, "Another one." *The nurse meant* "Another patient." *But the patient heard* her say something that meant "Are you pregnant again, you have enough children." A fruitful relationship never developed between this patient and nurses in the situation. A useful principle to bear in mind is: *in communicating with a new patient, who is also a stranger, try to say whatever it is that you wish the patient to hear.*

Another nursing situation points to a second principle. A public health nurse assigned to relieve in an area ordinarily covered by another nurse was assigned to locate a young girl, known to have had a venereal disease contact, who had failed to visit the physician and co-operate in treatment. On reaching the farm on which the girl lived the nurse encountered an enraged mother who felt that someone was trying to ruin her daughter's reputation. The nurse listened, joined in as conversation turned to farming and the difficulties in haying, and contributed an episode about meeting a bull en route to the farm. When the mother felt safer with the nurse, and was ready to listen, the nurse communicated the idea, "no one was trying to ruin your daughter but a check to be sure that she is all right means just one trip to the doctor for examination." When the nurse checked later with the physician she found that both mother and daughter had been in to see him. That is, they made use of the knowledge the nurse communicated to them. When nurses visit in homes it is always necessary for them to *accommodate to the direction of activity in the situation as they find it, await the development of good feeling, and then orient the family to the purpose of the visit and the services offered in a simple manner.* When a degree of identification is gained knowledge can be communicated and put to use; only where there is respect and mutual interest between two people can one person inform another.[2] Simple, clear, orienting statements about the situation and the reason for each being in it is a useful procedure and provides a basis for participant roles that may follow in the relationship. The individual is sick, this is a hospital, nurses are there to help the patient to meet his needs—these are a few of the things that can be said at the start of a relationship with a new patient.

Role of resource person

Nurses have functioned well as resource persons in situations where health information was needed. In this role, they viewed themselves as a source of supply on knowledge and technical procedures and they have taught much that was necessary for improving patient and community health. Nurses have always interpreted treatment plans and procedures in order to clarify "definitive care" rendered to patients.

A resource person provides specific answers to questions usually formulated with relation to a larger problem. Thus, a patient who has a medical problem might ask, "What is a normal body temperature?" and the nurse would cite the facts that inform the patient on this particular question. A patient might comment to a visiting nurse, "But, I don't know exactly how to change my dressings." The nurse might tell the patient how it could be done, demonstrate the procedure, and then observe and comment upon a return demonstration from the patient. Details related to a problem often raise questions that a professional expert can readily answer, out of a background of specialized preparation. Often

[2] Harry Stack Sullivan (M.D.), *Conceptions of Modern Psychiatry* (Washington, D.C., William Alanson White Psychiatric Foundation, 1947), pp. 46-48.

an individual in need does not have time to dig out facts useful to full understanding of a medical problem.

Patients frequently cast nurses into the role of resource person when this is not the role in which services can be most useful. A constant barrage of answers and advice can shut out a patient's wish to struggle with and think through his own problem. Competent nurses learn to discriminate opportunities to function in ways appropriate for constructive learning. The level of achievement a patient has reached is one criterion. Others include: the psychological readiness of the patient to grapple with difficulties that raise doubts, the psychological atmosphere in the situation, and the relevance of the question to illumination of the total problem. Nurses learn to make discriminating judgments in practice about questions that require direct, straightforward, factual answers and about those that involve feelings and may require application of principles of counseling.

Teaching roles

The role of teacher in nursing situations seems to be a combination of all of the roles discussed in this chapter. Teaching always proceeds from what the patient knows and it develops around his interest in wanting and being able to use additional medical information. Traditional teaching methods imply the acquisition of knowledge handed down by someone else and accepted on authority. The development of automatonlike habits is often an outcome. Learning through experience, which is the kind that nurses wish to promote, requires development of novel plans and situations that can unfold and lead to open-ended outcomes (i.e. outcomes which are unique products within this situation) that are fruitful for nurse and patient. A method that develops habits of grappling with difficulties that recur throughout life, a problem-solving approach in nursing, requires a variety of roles all of which constitute an aspect of teaching that is broadly conceived.

The role of leadership functions in nursing

Human endeavor, such as nursing, must portray leadership as a characteristic of democratic living. Leadership functions are demanded of nurses in local, national, and international situations. In clinical situations patient groups often cast nurses in the role of leader; individual patients identify with nurses and expect them to offer direction during the current difficulty.

Different kinds of leadership create different types of group atmosphere.[3] Democratic leadership encourages participation by everyone engaged in an endeavor: policies and goals are determined by all members; the agenda of work are shared by group decision; courses of action are planned in open discussion by members; all members are accepted as they are, interest being centered on the problem. The question can be raised: How democratic can *nursing practice* become? Democratic leadership in nursing situations implies that the patient will be permitted to be an active participant in designing nursing plans for him. Any nurse can attest that some patients could accept this responsibility at once while others would require infinite patience and a great deal more nursing time than is now made available in clinical situations. Democratic nursing is a goal to keep working toward.

In situations where autocratic leadership prevails, all policies, goals, and steps for their accomplishment are dictated by the leader. Symonds points out that blind identification with this kind of leadership occurs more readily in situations where individuals feel insecure and where their confidence in themselves is threatened.[4] In such situations patients often overvalue the nurse and substitute the nurse's goals and successes for their own wish to struggle. Fromm points out that

[3] P. L. Harriman (ed.), *Twentieth Century Psychiatry* (New York, Philosophical Library, Inc., 1946), pp. 200-30.
[4] Percival Symonds, *The Dynamics of Human Adjustment* (New York, Appleton-Century-Crofts, Inc., 1946), p. 335.

this tendency to give up one's feelings of independence and to gain strength by allying oneself with a stronger person is a mechanism of escape from freedom.[5] It is characterized by strivings for submission or domination, masochistic or sadistic strivings, that is, the acquired need to be hurt or to hurt others.

Nurses can learn to recognize overvaluation by patients, accept it as an aspect of the individual patient as he is, and yet accomplish the immediate tasks of nursing: *To be able to sit at the bedside of any patient, observe, and gather evidence on the way the patient views the situation confronting him, visualize what is happening inside the patient, as well as observe what is going on between them in the interpersonal relation.* Out of these data consideration of conditions required for health can be inferred. Providing assistance to the patient in meeting the tasks at hand requires a relationship of co-operation in which each can become aware, in some degree, of what those tasks are and how they can be met. Working with a patient in the solution of his problems requires democratic leadership if the experience is to lead to useful learning.

Nurses might well stop and ask themselves, in daily relations with others, what is being learned in this contact? Is the patient getting what I am saying, or is he taking in the way I am saying it? If one individual says something to another in a harsh, unfeeling manner does the other individual *catch* the content of what is said or the feeling tones that accompany it? Democratic leadership roles require attitudes of respect for the dignity and worth of each human being encountered and these attitudes cannot be assumed; they operate or they don't and the patient knows by way of his feelings what the attitudes of others are toward him.

Laissez-faire leadership leads to the development of another kind of group atmosphere. It is characterized by lack of active participation on the part of the individual in the

[5] Erich Fromm, *Escape from Freedom* (New York, Farrar & Rinehart, Inc., 1941), pp. 141-206.

leadership role; materials and information such as a resource role might provide are made available but the personality of the leader does not enter actively, except by default, into the interpersonal situation. As a rule, the laissez-faire leader neither interferes with or permits himself to be drawn into the activities around him. This kind of leader is not felt as a threat to the personalities in a group situation except as the lack of active interest is interpreted personally. Patients who rely upon nurses for concrete assistance only may not feel lacks in nurse-participation. Others who seek approbation as a way of expressing a need to strengthen their feeling of relatedness with others may be greatly deprived when materials are supplied but human interest is not shown. Showing interest in and respect for others in a way that is not interpreted as overpowering or absent is possible in democratic relations.

Leadership is a function in all situations. There are times when this role is fulfilled by other professional workers, or a patient may step in at an appropriate moment and aid a group to see new directions for activities under way. More often in nursing situations, however, it is the nurse whose professional skill can be utilized to indicate new possibilities and steps required for their actualization. The way in which these new directions can be identified, explored, and lead to new actions often depends upon how the nurse views this role and herself in it. The ability to function as a democratic leader is developed by participation in situations in the nursing school.

Surrogate roles

More frequently than is realized nurses are cast into surrogate roles by patients. That is, outside of his awareness the patient views the nurse as someone else; he does not see her as a person in her own way. One nurse may symbolize a mother figure, another may stand for a sibling, still another may personify some other cultural figure outside the family constellation—such as a teacher, another nurse met earlier in life, and the like. Instead of relating to the nurse as he finds her the patient is likely to relate to her in terms of the older relationship.

Substitute figures are raised in the mind of the patient when psychologically he is in a situation that reactivates feelings that were generated in a prior relationship. A patient who experiences feelings of helplessness, powerlessness, and strong wishes for dependency is required to use patterns of behavior that worked during periods when these feelings operated in a more natural setting, such as in infancy. The attitudes of the nurse, the feeling tones that she creates in the patient, the vehicles such as bathing that she uses influence the way in which the patient will view her. The behavior of the nurse—her appearance, mode of action, body gesture, manner of speaking—often operate to remind the patient of someone else. His relations with the nurse are more likely, then, to be in terms of his relations to that someone else he has in mind.

The nurse cannot control the mind of the patient. She cannot "remove" these illusory figures and compel the patient to recognize that she is not Aunt Martha, but Miss Jones. *A nurse can help patients to become aware of likenesses and differences and to come to know her as a person.*

Many nurses have had such experiences. The patient says, "You are the exact image of a teacher I once had." This provides the nurse with an opportunity for discovering how the patient views her—her behavior, her attitudes, her gestures, and the like. She can say, "I remind you of a teacher, I wonder what she was like." This opens communication and may lead the patient to a clarification of who the nurse is. On the other hand, if the nurse says, "A teacher, oh, no, I'd never want to be that," the patient may discern that he would offend the nurse if he reveals relationships that he feels exist between an earlier and this present situation. Communication in this area is cut off. The patient may persist and try again, later, saying, "You really do remind me of that school teacher that I was telling you about." This is to say, the patient feels there is now a closer relationship with the nurse and perhaps, "I can express my real feelings."

The values and feelings attached to the individual in the past life of the patient will color the expectations he has of the nurse who reminds him of the earlier figure. When those past experiences have included intense feelings of hostility, expected hindrances to personality expression, the patient is likely to reactivate and hence express these feelings toward the nurse. If the nurse *can accept the patient as he is* and can accept these expressed feelings as honest release of forces operating in the patient, he may stop and reflect on the differences between the nurse and the individual for whom she has stood. Previous behavior operated on a basis of likenesses, however fleeting and vague; present behavior can then begin to operate on the basis of an awareness of differences.

A nurse helps the patient to learn that there are likenesses and differences between people by being herself. The nursing profession and the basic school are concerned that each nurse will develop a wish to be useful to others in difficulty, to stand for the kind of person who is useful to the growth of others. A fledgling nurse, being herself in a situation, might get into interpersonal difficulties and require intervention of a competent graduate nurse supervisor who can aid the nurse and patient to work through the difficulties in a way fruitful for both parties. A student nurse who is not permitted to get into difficulties in any kind of situation may never develop awareness of self, such as is required by the tasks in nursing situations. A crisp, starched, technically expert automaton is one thing—a warmly human competent nurse always encounters difficulties in interpersonal relations and gradually develops her skill in recognizing and doing something to clarify understanding about them.

To the degree that a nurse is aware of her behavior, how she operates in her relations with others, she may be said to be herself. Nurses who are not so aware may view patients as illusory of individuals they have met in the past, and outside

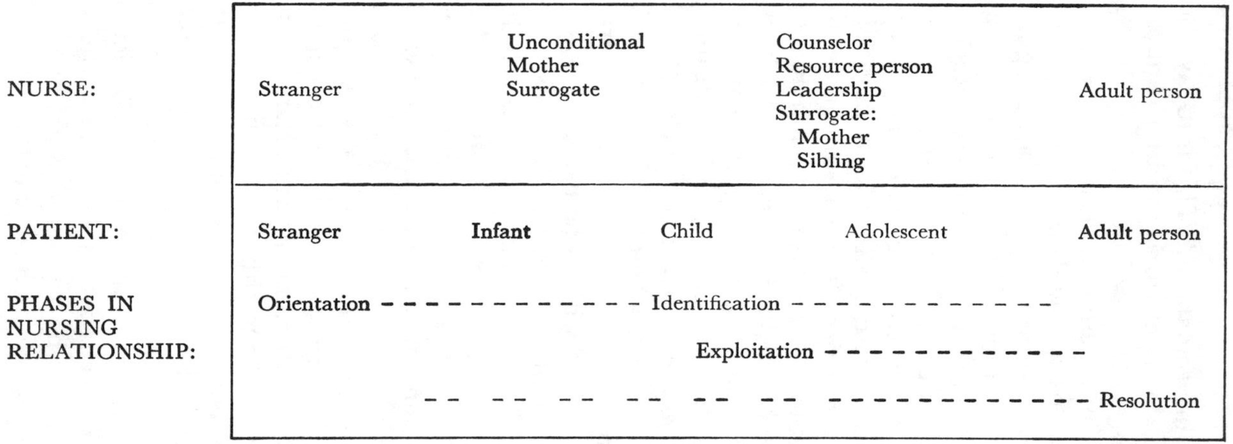

NURSE:	Stranger	Unconditional Mother Surrogate		Counselor Resource person Leadership Surrogate: Mother Sibling	Adult person
PATIENT:	Stranger	Infant	Child	Adolescent	Adult person
PHASES IN NURSING RELATIONSHIP:	Orientation – – – – – –	– – – – –	– – – Identification – – – – – – – – – – – – –	– – – – – –	– – – – – –
			Exploitation – – – – – – –	– – – – –	– – – – – Resolution

Fig. 5. Phases and changing roles in nurse-patient relationships.

of awareness relate to them on that basis. It is not uncommon to hear an occasional nurse refer to a patient as "mom," or, in another age group, as "sis." These patients are viewed as individuals that the nurse would like to think of and call by the names mom and sis. These are thought to be ways of addressing patients that show interest, affection, devotion. Actually, they cast the patient into roles that are not natural to the nursing situation and they demand nursing roles, such as child and sis, that are merely one aspect of what might be a total relationship. It is unrealistic to label the patient's role in a way that may defeat the development of person to person relationships. It is conceivable, too, that labeling the patient as mom denies that patient full recognition as an individual by classifying her under the stereotype of "mom."

The nurse and patient relationship moves on a continuum. At the point of first contact a patient might cast the nurse into the role of mother (or child, as the case may be). (See Fig. 5, p. 54.) If the patient is acutely ill, and requires continual mothering care, this surrogate role may be the logical one for the nurse to fulfill. However, each nurse has the responsibility for exercising her professional skill in aiding the relationship to move forward on the continuum, so that person to person relations compatible with chronological age levels can develop. *Surrogate roles are determined by psychological age factors that operate by reason of arrests in development, feelings that have been reactivated on the basis of illness, or demands made by individuals in a situation.*

A very ill patient may say, "I haven't been bathed by someone else since I was a baby." The nurse might reply, "Yes, when you are sick like this I know that you must feel somewhat like a baby." The patient may respond later with, "You remind me of my mother. She used to be that fussy about getting my ears clean." The nurse might respond to this remark, which gives her clues about areas she may be stressing that were overstressed in childhood, by saying, "Yes, I guess nurses do seem like mothers to patients when they are real sick." Or, she might say, "You feel as if you are being mothered again, as a child might feel." *These ways of re-sponding, which do not impose goals that the nurse has in mind about how patients should feel, aid the patient in becoming aware of what is actually felt during the experi-ence.*

Later in the relationship, as the patient's condition im-proves, he may offer to help himself, saying, "Nurse, why don't you give me that washcloth and let me do my face and ears." The nurse, recognizing this as a "growth cue" or a step toward interdependence, might respond, "You want to begin to do things for yourself. Here is the washcloth; it's all ready for your part of the job." *The relationship has moved from one in which mother and child surrogate roles operated to one in which both parties are beginning to function as adults capable of defining areas of independence and areas of interdependence.*

Consider what practical difference it might make if the following responses were used. Suppose that the patient said, "You remind me of my sister; she was always trying to boss me around," and the nurse responded with, "I am only carry-ing out what the doctor ordered." What might happen to communication between nurse and patient? Would it be facilitated or cut off? Suppose that a patient said, "If you will hand me that washcloth I will take care of my face and ears," and the nurse replied, "You are too sick to do that; I am the nurse and I am supposed to bathe you." A patient acutely ill and greatly in need of psychological mothering is told, "Here is a basin of water; wash yourself." What hap-pens to the feelings of the patient?

Or, consider the case in some hospitals where nurses are required to bathe patients until they are convalescent, after which they may go to the bathroom and do a part of the bath-ing for themselves. When the patient has completed his part of the job the nurse says, "Now, get into bed and I will wash your feet." The patient remonstrates, "But they are not dirty. I did as much as I could but, honestly, they couldn't be very dirty." The nurse replies, "In this hospital there is a rule: all patients must have their feet washed every day." What mixed feelings are generated in this patient who is expected and is able to take care of himself, and then is shown that he is not entirely able?

These responses to remarks that patients make are not offered as rules for conduct. They are meant to show one way in which a patient could be permitted to experience his own feelings and be helped to become aware of what those feelings are. Conduct in nursing situations cannot be decided by anyone except each nurse operating in the situation. As each nurse examines her attitudes toward people she comes to recognize her philosophy of life and the principles that guide her behavior in life situations. As each nurse develops skill in observation and in understanding the situation as it is seen by the patient, appropriate nursing actions will flow out of such understanding.

Permitting the patient to re-experience older feelings in new situations of helplessness, but with professional acceptance and attention that provokes personality development, requires a relationship in which the nurse recognizes and responds in a variety of surrogate roles. When older experiences are relived and re-examined in a new situation a reorganization of experience can take place. Re-experiencing complete helplessness, and mothering care in relation to it, may mean that the patient feels like an infant; this role may be followed by reactivation of childlike feelings, then adolescent difficulties that have not been worked through with a mothering person, before the patient reaches full expression of adult needs. The nurse requires understanding of the mother role, as it moves on a continuum from unconditional acceptance and attention through all its phases toward a person to person relationship. However, at certain points in the relationship the patient may cast the nurse in a sibling role, working through unsolved difficulties in relations with brothers or sisters, with her or with a group of patients, and then return her to the mother role. *Perception of the role in which the patient casts the nurse, identification of the difficulty that is being worked through, and sustaining a working re-lationship that develops awareness in the patient of how he feels are nursing skills.*

Concrete experiences, such as taking food, accepting medi-cations, permitting a nurse to bathe him, undergoing treat-ments, around which cluster the patient's most deeply perceived human feelings provide opportunities for express-ing and finding out what is felt about mothering. Experi-ences, such as living in a ward with other patients, sharing a nurse or a doctor, sharing facilities available for all, often give rise to opportunities to discover and reorient feelings about siblings. Room, ward, and hospital boundaries, which limit the freedom of movement of a patient, and restrictions on visitors, telephone calls, and the like offer experiences in expressing and finding out about relations to persons in au-thority. The challenge in nursing practice is in making these learning experiences count in terms of recovery from an ill-ness or operation as well as in terms of further development of personality.

The patient's earlier experiences in life will determine the impressions and expectations he will have about nurses. Older relationships with women and men will be expressed in his anticipation of what the nurse will be able to do with him in the current situation. Earlier experiences are often decisive as to whether he will be able readily to accept the ministrations of women or men nurses or whether the need for care will embarrass him. If the patient has had congenial relations in the past—useful in terms of full expression of his evolving personality—he will probably meet the nurse with positive expectations. If, in the past, his experiences have included getting advice that he could use, from a per-son who respected and liked him, it will be easier for him to accept advice from the nurse at the outset. However, if the mother of the patient has been inconsiderate and demanding, and the feelings generated by her authoritarian attitudes were reinforced in relations with nurses, teachers, and neighbors who were also autocratic the patient may expect that the nurse will relate to him in the same way. In fact, he may feel most insecure if she does not. He may seek or demand orders from her, in order to rebel against them. He may refuse to co-operate, rebel against advice, withhold needed information about his present problem, as a way of showing his contempt for persons who seem to have authority over him.

Patients who have worked through their feelings and difficulties in relations with parents so that as adults they relate to parents as adults rather than as children may have few difficulties in coming to know and to use nurses and nursing. Mature adults are those who have willingly put aside childlike needs for a mother person and are able to function as full-grown persons. A social situation illustrates what is meant. A mother who felt that she needed to overprotect her daughter always functioned toward her in an unconditional way—washing her clothes and ironing them, preparing all meals, calling her each morning to go to work, deciding on clothes that could be purchased, deciding on what she should wear. After her daughter married and subsequently had a child of her own, she came to spend a two-week vacation with her mother. On arrival, the mother took complete charge of the infant, the laundry, the cooking, and all details connected with the visit. In other words, the relationship lapsed to the earlier mother and child one in which the daughter was freed from all adult responsibility. This relationship was not precipitated by a crisis; it had never developed beyond what can be seen in the evidence presented. A person-to-person relationship on an adult level requires active participation of all parties in planning and carrying out the work required by a situation.

In nursing situations, the complex relationship undergoes further change when the doctor enters the field. How nurse and doctor feel about each other, their capacities for deeply felt mutual respect, determine the solidarity of their efforts. How the nurse feels about men in authority, how the doctor feels about women functioning co-operatively with him in situations that carry authority of their own, what the patient perceives and expects from each and their relations with one another—all make a difference in the outcome. Facilitating changes and improvements in understanding and resolving the difficulty faced by the patient with professional help requires collaboration based upon attitudes of trust in and respect for the capacity of each to grow and change. When professional education demands conventional attitudes and does not provide for expression and examination of genuine underlying feelings, collaborative relations are difficult to establish. When a nurse looks to the doctor as a father or when the doctor looks upon the nurse as a sister or an unconditional mother, without being aware of feelings that motivate these views that operate in the situation, mature professional relationships cannot be established. When the patient casts the nurse into the role of mother and simultaneously casts the doctor into the role of father, viewing himself as the child in this surrogate family constellation, it is necessary for the professional persons to recognize the operation of this triad relationship. There is a unit relationship and separate relations toward the patient; these relationships are selectively determined by the patient on the basis of earlier family relations and are called out by his present feelings. A new family experience may be felt below awareness by the patient.

The challenge in nursing practice is that of developing learning experiences for patients that make use of their separate relations with them; collaboration with physicians aims at the development of similarly useful experiences that make use of the unit relationship. The focus is upon the presenting medical problem, the unfolding interpersonal situation, the day-by-day difficulties that arise in relation to nursing care, in a way that helps the patient to develop his personality and to use his capacities in a more mature way than he did before he became ill. This requires recognition of the roles in which the patient casts the nurse, and of the roles in which the nurse casts the patient without consciously knowing it, and the development of awareness of changing roles as the relationship moves toward a more adult one. It requires recognition that roles may shift momentarily, that others entering the field may be invested with family roles, that the patient may be unable to relinquish a role until his needs as he feels them are met and recognized in awareness. Respect for the individual as he is always includes the possibility that he will err, trust that he will profit from his mistakes, and belief that given sufficient experiences and evidence out of which new skills can develop that he will move in that direction. Surrogate roles are determined by psychological needs; they give rise to psychological tasks to be met in nursing situations by nurses.[6]

Role of counselor

The processes of self-renewal, self-repair, self-awareness arise within the individual. The purposeful behavior these processes make possible are initiated by the self. Interpersonal conditions in the situation can often be improved so that the responding patient will want to discover his problems and reveal the difficulties he faces, to himself and others, rather than to suppress or distort them. As Wertheimer has pointed out, individuals learn only as they re-create the steps, re-experience the feelings, and view their difficulties in new perspective.[7] Facilitating these self-directed actions are counseling functions.

All counseling functions in nursing are determined by the purpose of all nurse-patient relationships, namely, the *promotion* of experiences leading to health. This purpose is achieved through a series of more immediate objectives. Helping a patient to become aware of conditions required for health, providing these conditions whenever possible,

[6] See Part III.

[7] Max Wertheimer, *Productive Thinking* (New York, Harper & Brothers, 1945), pp. 191-95.

aiding him to identify threats to health, and using the evolving interpersonal event to facilitate learning—are all steps in the achievement of purpose.

In view of round-the-clock relations with patients and the changing roles and variety of essential services that are required, a nurse cannot function as counselor in the same manner as a psychotherapist or nondirective counselor. The therapist has, usually, a specific place in which therapeutic sessions are conducted, a specific hour that is assigned to a patient, and developed techniques that are used to identify and illuminate a central, interpersonal difficulty that a patient faces and that has wide ramifications in his relations with others. The therapist can function in passive or neutral ways, devoting the full therapeutic hour to the patient as he wishes to use it or as the therapist deems necessary. Moreover, the therapist can elect techniques that he will use. All techniques fall on a continuum from direct approaches, progressively less direct ones, to nondirective methods for helping patients to gain insight into their difficulties.[8]

What then is the therapeutic, or counseling role, in nursing? How is it determined? What purposes does it serve? What skills does it require? Can nurses function in this role under present organization of nursing service? Are administrative changes indicated? These questions when discussed by nurses in particular situations provide leads for designing a framework and method of procedure for using counseling roles, into which patients often cast nurses.

Since nurses must provide many other essential services, they have a more active role in the therapeutic endeavor than other therapists. We have already defined therapy, in this work, as a relationship that provides satisfaction for needs unmet in the past through which continuing growth becomes possible. Experiences that patients undergo and that compel actions of one kind or another—such as anxiety, doubt, frus-

[8] In this connection see: D. Ewen Cameron, "Behavioral Concepts and Psychotherapy," Psychiatric Quarterly, Utica State Hospital Press, New York, 24:227-242 (April, 1950).

tration, conflict, and guilt—are to be discussed in Part II. Psychological tasks that arise in nursing situations, the handling of which have direct bearing upon the possibility of further personality development, will be developed in detail in Part III. Here we are concerned with the identification of principles that might govern the counseling role as it interlocks with all roles previously discussed in this chapter.

Counseling in clinical situations has to do with the *way* in which nurses respond to demands made upon them, rather than to what those demands are. The process is largely one of expanding experiences dimly intelligible to the patient at first, so that they become better understood by patient and nurse. Experiences that have to do with *how the patient feels about himself,* as a person who is ill, as a worker who has just had that part of his body amputated that is vital to continuing his chosen work, as a parent whose children might suffer because he has a long-term illness. Frequently, a social worker can be helpful to the patient's family in making suitable arrangements that ease the pressure upon the patient, but *how he feels about what is happening to him*—about being dependent upon others to exercise their power in behalf of his responsibilities—requires counseling roles on the part of nurses.

The way in which the patient views himself and the experience of being sick, as it has actually been undergone from the first impression through a multitude of detailed, related experiences at the hands of nurses and others, makes a difference in whether it will be dissociated, disconnected from awareness, or whether it will be integrated into the backlog of other useful experiences he has had in life. Patients *dissociate experiences that cannot be permitted or remembered in awareness. More often, the feelings connected with the experience are pushed out of awareness, the event itself being subject to recall or actively remembered.* Dissociation may be an active tendency, which the patient has used consistently throughout life, or it may be one that is forced into operation by requirements in a new situation from which the patient cannot escape. *Counseling in nursing has to do with helping the patient to remember and to understand fully what is happening to him in the present situation, so that the experience can be integrated with rather than dissociated from other experiences in life.* Two examples illustrate what is meant:

Anne was an aggressive six-year-old who continuously asserted, "Oh, I love my mother, I love her more than anyone else in the world, I love her more than she loves me. I love her so much it hurts and I hate to go to school and leave her." Sensing that this child was expressing conventional attitudes and that her real feelings about her mother had been selectively not attended or dissociated, the observer used a social visit to help this child to examine her feelings. A nondirective method was used.

On arrival, Anne climbed upon the desk and asserted to the observer sitting on the divan, "I'm going to jump on you."

O: You plan to jump on me?

A: Yes, I am going to jump on you. You'd better watch out!

O: You want me to watch out, because you are going to jump on me?

A: Yes, here I come, I'm going to jump on you!

O: You're planning to jump on me?

A: Will you hit me if I jump on you?

O: You want to know whether I will hit you if you jump on me?

A: Yes, will you? Here I come, are you going to hit me?

O: You'd like to know whether I will hit you if you jump on me?

A: Yes, will you? I said, will you hit me?

O: You would really like to know if I will hit you if you hit me, by jumping on me?

A: (screaming) I said, will you? I have to know. *Will you hit me if I jump?*

O: You must know before you jump whether I shall hit you?

A: Tell me. Tell me. Are you going to hit me back if I jump on you?

O: You think I might hit back if you jump on me?

A: Yes, yes, that's what my mother does. She always hits me and says mean things to me when I do things. And last night I dreamed about my schoolteacher and she hit me when I threw a bottle out of the window. And I think you will hit me, too.

O: You think that all women might hit you back when you hurt them?

A: I have to know, I have to know. Are you going to hit me?

O: You really have to know before you hit, whether others will hurt you back.

A: Yes, I have to know. I know my mother will hit me. And I have to know whether you will.

O: You want to know whether all women are exactly like your mother?

A: Yes, will you hit me like she does? She always hits me. She makes me angry. She says things and does things that make me angry.

O: You would like to know whether all women will say things that make you angry—before you hurt them?

A: I guess I'll just jump and find out. (Whereupon she jumped and, of course, the observer did not hit. Anne then asked for a story, this being a pleasant pattern in previous relationships with the observer.)

O: What shall the story be about?

A: Tell it about a little boy and he had a garden and his mother and a man came and planted some grass and the boy dug up the grass and his mother hit him and then she said he could dig up the whole yard if he wanted to, that it was spoiled now.

Recognizing the fact that the boy was Anne and that the situation was an experience that she had actually undergone, the observer made up a story around the theme of ambivalence. A discussion followed during which other feelings of love and hatred for her mother were identified and to some extent clarified.

Here is a social situation in which a nurse functioned as counselor during one unit in the total experience, with some delineation of the source of ambivalence and some relaxation of the tendency to selectively inattend or dissociate the intense hatred that was felt toward her mother. The situation was developed so that it was possible to pass from one aspect of the relationship that was specifically therapeutic counseling to one that was social in nature.

A second example illustrates dissociating tendencies at work in an individual who had been operated for radical mastectomy. In conversation, fifteen years later, the following evidence is gathered:

"I went swimming the other day. I used to enjoy swimming, in fact I am a pretty good swimmer, but my 'cups' kept falling down, and I felt embarrassed. I didn't enjoy it the way I used to do. You know, I had a radical mastectomy fifteen years ago, but it never bothered me until lately. In fact, I never thought of it—even while I was in the hospital—I was so anxious to get back to my work and all. I never gave it a thought but about a year ago I had a routine physical examination, and the physician said, 'That was quite a large operation, you must have experienced considerable psychic trauma.' But, I told her, as a matter of fact I didn't, I didn't mind it at all. Then a few months ago I attended an institute and I thought of it there—in more or less fleeting fashion. But, lately, I have found myself thinking of it a great deal and when I do, I cry and think to myself—why can't you be like other people."

It can be seen from the evidence presented that this patient did not experience her real feelings about this surgical destruction of a part of her, at the time of operation. This is partly because an active dissociating tendency was then in operation, on her part, and perhaps, too, nurses did not promote expression of feelings connected with the event. *To help this patient to experience in awareness her real feelings connected with the event at the time of operation was a counseling function.* The feelings that were not experienced in awareness were pushed underground but nevertheless operated to distort her enjoyment of life and her relations with people; feelings that are recognized and examined in awareness can be put aside willingly as plans for accepting life as it is are made.

When patients say, "I am worried about that operation to-morrow," they are initiating a discussion about feelings connected with it. If the nurse says, "You have some worried feelings about the operation," she leaves the door open for further communication of what the patient feels. If she says, "There, there, you have nothing to worry about. The doctor will take care of everything," the patient's feelings connected with the anticipated event are denied expression—they must either be worked through by the patient, alone, or be disso-ciated from awareness. Moreover, the feeling of powerless-ness that is connected with putting oneself in the hands of a surgeon and nurses is reinforced when the patient cannot find out what his real worries are. *It is not a simple matter to consent psychologically to manipulation or partial destruc-tion of one's own body and yet integrate the event as one experience in life among many from which something valu-able has been learned.* This task faced by the patient requires professional nursing counseling. Even though the patient has discussed it with his surgeon, when he comes face to face with the operations preparatory to surgical intervention new feel-ings arise and need to be worked through as his abdomen is being scrubbed, painted, and prepared for the operation.

Medical problems and surgical operations that have to do with the erogenous zones—oral, anal, and genital areas—re-

quire full psychological preparation.[9] This principle implies that tonsillectomies, circumcisions, and hemorrhoidectomies, while minor operations from the standpoint of physical risk involved, are major ones from the point of view of the psychological meaning to the patient.

Careful preparation includes assisting the patient to identify, to formulate, and to accept his real feelings about the surgical event to be undergone; to understand its meaning to him, and yet to move forward toward the goal to be achieved. When pathology concerning the oral, anal, and genital areas is involved the role of the patient's feelings and full consent are of paramount importance for full integration and acceptance of this event as one actually occurring to the patient. Patients who say, "I didn't mind it a bit"; "I didn't feel a thing"; "I hardly remember that I had the operation," are ones about whom a nurse might well ask herself: Has he dissociated this event? What long-term effect on his total functioning will his present attitude have?

It cannot be taken for granted that the patient will be able to appreciate fully the significance of the operation without professional assistance. This is equally true of dental work, all rectal procedures, such as enemas, and genital intervention such as surgery or pelvic examination. These zones of interaction—oral, anal, genital—have had considerable weight in character formation; satisfaction has been achieved and anxiety expressed and often relieved through their varied use in the life history of the patient. Getting clear on what is felt and what the experience means to him are the only safeguards against psychic trauma occurring during a particular experience.

How the nurse accomplishes the tasks outlined above, what counseling techniques she uses in her relations with patients, will depend largely upon her philosophy about people and techniques that she selects to be compatible with that philosophy. Many textbooks are now available on coun-

[9] William A. White, *Twentieth Century Psychiatry* (New York, W. W. Norton & Company, Inc., 1936), p. 78.

seling that aid nurses to identify techniques compatible with their attitudes and beliefs. Some basic principles can be cited:

Observation precedes interpretation of the collected data.[10] *If* giving advice is to be used as a technique in counseling, careful observation and skillful listening always precede the giving of advice. When nurses develop and use a technique of listening that is largely nondirective and nonmoralizing the patient will *gradually discover* facets about himself that he did not recognize before; a series of such discoveries in the course of any illness may for some patients prove illuminating and therapeutic.[11] When the nurse confronts the patient with some "truth" about himself as she has interpreted it, the patient may experience severe anxiety, panic, or rage.[12] Patients can discover and use new insights that refer to the self when they are given the lead in determining whether they wish to reveal feelings and underlying problems that serve to distort their relations with others in the situation. Nursing provides conditions and methods under which each patient can become a more productive person. The principles, or preconceptions, that guide counseling roles are determined by the personality of the nurse and the knowledge that has been brought to bear and reshaped it during her basic professional education.[13]

Summary

Roles that are demanded of nurses arise during interpersonal relations with individuals or communities. Some specific ones have been discussed. Other roles, such as consultant, tutor, safety agent, mediator, administrator, recorder, ob-

[10] See Part IV for full discussion on observation.
[11] Carl Rogers, *Counseling and Psychotherapy* (New York, Houghton Mifflin Company, 1942).
[12] Lawrence S. Kubie, *The Nature of Psychotherapy,* Bulletin of the New York Academy of Medicine, Vol. 19, No. 3 (March, 1943), pp. 183-194.
[13] Sullivan, *op. cit.,* pp. 46-48, 94.

server, and researcher or study-maker have been left to the intelligence and imagination of the reader. Observation and recording, as methods, are discussed in Part IV. Some of these roles are always determined in the situation; guiding principles can be formulated in advance and expanded in the process of taking various roles in situations.[14] Nurses often symbolize nonrational roles to patients, that is, they stand for but are not mothers of patients, and they take on these roles at the same time helping the patient to clarify his preconceptions and to become aware of the nurse as a person, in her own right. Person-to-person relationships depend upon these prior steps in the nursing process. While some patients may immediately develop person to person relations with nurses, knowing in awareness what they expect of them, many of them move through a series of roles as the relationship develops. Nursing situations and relationships of nurse to patient are not administered at present so that any one role can operate without interlocking with another. It is conceivable that when nursing service is structured, so that disciplinary and administrative functions are centered in the supervisor or head nurse, who then oversees that all persons in the ward situation are governed by the limits and boundaries hospital administration requires, that staff nurses may be left free for a more fluid, permissive, therapeutic relationship. Nevertheless, nursing roles will always overlap in some degree and require that nurses identify the authority in the situation that demands taking one or another role.[15] Skill in taking roles as outlined above is developed in practice in nursing situations under competent supervision.

[14] George H. Mead, *Mind, Self and Society* (University of Chicago Press, Chicago, 1934). *See also* Theodore M. Newcomb, *Social Psychology* (New York, The Dryden Press, 1950).

[15] Mary Parker Follett, *Dynamic Administration* (New York, Harper & Brothers, 1942). Perhaps one of the most significant and helpful texts on principles of group dynamics as they affect organization and leadership in action. Uses the word "task-authority" to show that each situation generates its own tasks carrying their own authority.

Part II. INFLUENCES IN NURSING SITUATIONS

Purpose: *The purpose of Part II is to identify those psychobiological experiences that influence the functioning of personalities. Needs, frustration, conflict, and anxiety all provide energy that is transformed into some form of action. Understanding what these experiences are, which compel destructive or constructive responses from nurses and patients, is a step in the direction of personal and rational control of behavior. These psychobiological experiences that energize people and demand movement in interpersonal relations will be discussed and related to experiences that arise in clinical situations. These understandings will then provide a basis for discussion of psychological tasks in nursing, as presented in Part III.*

CHAPTER 4

Human Needs

Overview

THE FUNCTION of personality is to grow and and to develop. Nursing is a process that seeks to facilitate development of personality by aiding individuals to use those compelling forces and experiences that influence personality in ways that ensure maximum productivity. Nurses are assistants and helpers, rather than manipulators of people; they seek to aid individuals and communities in providing and using suitable conditions that will meet their needs. Everyone has needs that are instinctual ones or that have been acquired in the process of socialization. Primary or acquired needs that are met in one situation, in some degree, arise again in new situations. In each situation that an individual finds himself needs arise; when needs that are uppermost are met the tension they create subsides until other needs are activated. The purpose of this chapter is to aid in identification of needs that arise in nursing situations, to clarify how they affect the setting and achieving of goals in interpersonal relations.

Essential questions

What kinds of basic human needs seek expression in nursing situations? How are they expressed? What happens when needs are not met? What are mature, professional attitudes toward needs that patients demonstrate in their behavior? How can a nurse find out what are the psychological needs of patients? How can a nurse meet those needs and still complete all of the work that has been assigned to her for a given morning? Is it important to pay attention to the needs of patients? Aren't professional persons like nurses better able to decide what a patient needs? These questions lead into a discussion of nursing situations from which generalizations can be made and principles stated when confirmed in many situations. Two clinical experiences are outlined to provide a basis for discussion of needs as they affect the learning that is possible in a nursing situation.

Clinical Analysis No. 1

A NINE-YEAR-OLD BOY TACKLES A MEDICAL PROBLEM

Steps in the learning experience:	Behavior observed:
A course of action is demanded by an emergent problem.	The presence of forty-two unsightly warts on the boy's arms and leg initiated a decision on what to do about them.
A course of action is decided upon.	Participation in discussion with his parents led to a decision to remove the warts; an appointment was made to visit a physician in his office.
A goal is set. (Note the need to be like others, to be without warts.)	Anticipation of removal of the warts was expressed by the boy, "I will be glad when mine are gone."
As the course of action is pursued, the experience is evaluated by the boy so that what is happening can be understood.	En route to the physician's office the boy asked, "Will it hurt?" (to the nurse). "Did you have warts off?"
(Note the need to share the experience, to get information, to feel safe.)	(In response to her affirmative reply.) "How long did it take to get well? How many is a few?"
	(In the physician's office) "Why does the doctor want my pants off? What are you (physician) going to do? Can I see?"

Steps in the learning experience:

Behavior observed:

Appropriate emotions arise to show how he feels about what is happening.

(Note the need to like himself, to feel pride and pleasure in accomplishment of part of the goal.)

Upon sitting up to watch the doctor remove the warts, the boy noted that the largest one was removed, then a smaller one. The boy *smiled.* When the number to be removed that day was completed the boy was *grinning* and seemed *pleased.* He went to meet his mother and told her all about the event with a great deal of *pride.*

The experience moves on to the next phase; a next task emerges and demands accomplishment.

(Note the need to participate in setting subgoals.)

The experience continues until the desired satisfactory goal is reached or until a new attainable goal is set up.

Since all forty-two warts could not be removed in one day the boy was asked to make another appointment. The physician suggested the next Tuesday or Wednesday. The boy spoke up and said, "Tuesday." The goal that leads to *satisfaction,* in this observable event, is the removal of the unsightly warts. This is the goal of the boy, the doctor, the parents, and the nurse —all of whom participate in this event in the accomplishment of the goal.

The goal or outcome is accepted.

Clinical Analysis No. 2

A Twenty-two-year-old Male Struggles to Avoid a Medical Problem

Steps in the experiential process:

Behavior observed:

A course of action is demanded by an emergent problem.

The patient's mother brought him to a clinic for an initial visit, one year ago, where a diagnosis of "moderately advanced tuberculosis of one lung" was made. The patient was interviewed by a social worker and then hospitalized.

*Steps in the experiential
process:*

Behavior observed:

Later, the patient was referred to a public health nurse who made a home visit.

A course of action is decided upon.

(Note the need to rebel against goals set by others for him, the need to be at home.)

The hospitalization—as a course of action—was decided upon by clinic authorities and the patient's mother. The patient had refused treatment during the interview with the social worker; following hospitalization he had "escaped" and then returned home. The patient's course of action was to remain at home.

A goal is set.

(Note the need for self-assertion, for mastery over the situation, for hurting himself in order to meet prior needs.)

To the nurse the patient asserted, "I better tell you that I am not going there any more. Not even if I die."

As the course of action is pursued the experience is evaluated so that what is happening can be understood.

(Note the need to show power against the family who exploited him to meet their needs at an earlier date.)

During the interview the patient blamed his mother for being responsible for his illness. He had explained to the social worker that she made him work since he was a child to support the whole family—his father was dead—and now that his sisters were earning money they all wanted him out of the house. So, his mother had brought him for examination with the idea of sending him to the hospital.

Appropriate emotions arise to show how he feels about what is happening.

(Note the need to belong to his family, to gain recognition from them, and to defeat them in sending him away.)

(Note the need to project blame on the house, rather than the organisms in his lung.)

(Note a need for someone to intervene for him; to show him

The patient asserted to the nurse, "I feel bad."

"All of them are ashamed that I am sick."

"It is very hot in bed. The roof is too low. That heat gives me fever."

"Please talk to mother about the roof."

"You can come anytime you want. I am always here."

(This latter remark indicates the strength of his goal to remain

*Steps in the experiential
process:*

interest and respect as a person.)

The experience moves on to the
next phase; a next task emerges
and demands accomplishment.

(Note that the nurse does not
insinuate other needs—such as the
need for hospitalization—but prepares to meet the needs that are
emergent so that more mature
ones can arise.)

(Note how the nurse plays into
the patient's need for attention
from his family not by verbalizing
sympathy but by defining concrete
tasks they can perform for him
as well as to protect themselves.)

(Later, she will aid the patient
to resolve these dependent family
ties, as interdependent relations
with family members develop.)

The experience continues until
the desired goal is reached or
until a new, attainable goal is set
up.

Behavior observed:

home, and it connotes initial willingness to identify with the nurse.)
The nurse began to define the
home situation as one in which
he could begin treatment.

"I think the best thing for you
is to stay in bed. The room can
be made cooler by putting a sheet
of paperboard right under the
zinc of the roof. You have a good
view through the windows. You
can read, too, when you are not
very tired. You need not turn to
spit in that bowl; it is easier if
you spit in paper napkins like
this (demonstrates) and put them
in a paper bag pinned to your
bedside. Then they can be burned
and the germs are sure to be
killed. I will talk to your mother.
She can fold the napkins and make
the bags for you."

(To the nurse as she was leaving)
"Please bring me an old copy of
a newspaper when you come."

(Interest in a new goal may be
developing as the patient shows
the nurse his dependence upon
her and his awareness of her interest in him.)

The nursing tasks in future relations included:

Assisting the patient to review and
redefine his present set goal. Assisting his family to recognize,
accept, and meet the patient's
needs for recognition and belonging in ways that permit him to
grow. Assisting the patient to
clarify his view of himself so that
he can prefer to deal with his
medical problem in a rational
manner.

Discussion of human needs

A summary of needs expressed in the two foregoing experiences might help in making generalizations about them:

The nine-year-old boy	*The twenty-two-year-old male*
To be like others.	To rebel against goals set by others.
To be without warts.	
To share experiences.	To be at home although ill.
To get information.	To assert self.
To feel safe with the doctor.	To show mastery over the situation.
To like himself.	
To feel pride and pleasure.	To hurt self, as a way of defeating others.
To participate in setting subgoals.	
	To show personal power.
	To belong to the family.
	To project blame onto objects.
	To express dependence on the nurse.
	To have the nurse's interest.

Looking at the sequence of needs emergent in these two situations it can be seen that the boy seems to have *two overall goals:* satisfaction of his needs and wants in the achievement of his goals and security, specifically, at the point where what was happening in his relations with the doctor was not clear to him. The patient, on the other hand, behaves in ways that are designed to make him feel safe. His goals are *not* set *in terms of what he wants, what can lead to satisfaction of rational desires,* but rather are oriented to *what he does not want, what makes him feel safe and secure.* The boy's experience gives the *feeling that he is for something, that his behavior is oriented to goals that are out in front of him.* The patient's data give the *feeling that he is compelled to be against almost everything, that his goals are oriented to something he has been deprived of in the past.*

Sullivan defines these two "end-states," of satisfaction and of security, as the over-all goals in interpersonal relations and shows how performances, such as seen in the patients' experiences above, are mainly "security operations."[1] Symonds refers to two main purposes of each organism as "self-maintenance" and the "perpetuation of the species."[2] Self-maintenance, security operations, survival, isolationism are all terms that describe actions that are calculated to help an individual to feel safe, to feel that he will not die—literally or figuratively. Satisfaction, perpetuation of the species, participation in the ongoing stream of civilization, extension of the self into the community, interdependence are words that denote performances that have to do with affirmation and fulfillment of man's wants, goals, and desires so that new goals can be set and achieved by and for all of the people. These words connote literal death as a natural condition of life that moves onward.

Many workers have defined and prepared lists of human needs or wishes. Thomas suggests four main directive impulses: desires for security, for new experience, for affectional responses, and for recognition.[3] Healy, and others, have suggested a fifth drive, the wish for mastery.[4] Rosenzweig suggests criteria for classification of needs, showing how they fall on a continuum: needs for protection of the organism against dysfunctioning; needs that permit expression of growth levels; reproductive and thus, self-expansive needs; and needs in which creative activities are biologically and symbolically expressed in behavior.[5] Symonds refers to a list of principles that clarify physiological functioning as it underlies psychological drives.[6] These principles may be summarized as follows: *When immediate needs are met more mature needs arise. Needs create tension; they may but do*

[1] Sullivan, *op. cit.*, p. 6.

[2] Symonds, *op. cit.*, p. 12.

[3] W. I. Thomas, *The Unadjusted Girl* (New York, Little, Brown & Company, 1925), pp. 1-40.

[4] William Healy, *Personality in Formation and Action* (New York, W. M. Norton & Co., Inc., 1938), p. 78.

[5] J. McV. Hunt (ed.), *Personality and the Behavior Disorders* (New York, The Ronald Press Company, 1944), Ch. XI, p. 381.

[6] Symonds, *op. cit.*, Ch. II.

not always give rise to anxiety. All behavior aims to reduce tension arising from needs. When a strong need is uppermost, all behavior is directed toward it and other needs may be unrecognized. Most actions involve a fusion of several needs or drives. Symonds also asserts that *satisfaction of present needs is a guarantee of meeting deprivations of them more effectively in the future.*[7]

The last principle stated above probably accounts for those patients who are able to endure delays and to await attention to their needs, when ill, without becoming demanding of nurses or withdrawing entirely from the situation; their needs have been satisfied in the past and consequently they are able to use the tension to recognize reality factors in nursing service limitations. These patients do not present crucial challenges to nursing service; those patients who require assistance in order to meet present needs and to develop their personalities further require personalized nursing that makes use of psychological and social science principles in designing nursing plans for them.

Maslow points out that maladjustments and neuroses are dominated by basic needs that have been unmet in the past, showing that the *healthy* person is one who since his basic needs have been met can be further motivated to develop and actualize his highest potentialities.[8] In the same vein, experiences with illness during which basic needs are expressed together with feelings of helplessness and powerlessness experienced in earlier years can be used for providing a foundation for further actualization of capacities.

Needs create tension and tension creates energy that is transformed into some form of behavior. (See Fig. 6, p. 81.) Patients often find relief from tension through nail biting, scratching, hoarding food and soap, using biting and cynical words, and the like. Some patients use their tension and its energy to demand attention from nurses and *this is probably*

---

[7] *Ibid.,* p. 43.

[8] A. H. Maslow, "A Theory of Human Motivation," *Psychological Review,* 50:370-396 (July, 1943).

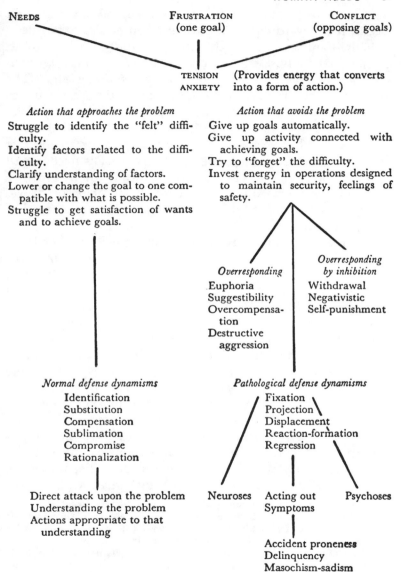

Fig. 6.   Psychological experiences that provide energy that is
transformed into various forms of behavior.

a more direct approach to the problem of meeting their needs; it is rewarding to the patient when needs are satisfied.[9] When infants suck their thumbs, or children are enuretic, pediatricians advise their mothers to *ignore the symptoms and meet the child's needs for affection and attention.* The principle is the same in handling behavior that adults use to relieve tension, such as ringing the call bell frequently, complaining about nurses, hoarding food and soap, and the like. Identifying what needs are emergent that are not being met in the situation and planning to supply what is needed will make it possible for patients to put aside their excessive demands. Anticipating the needs of the patient leaves the patient free to use the tension that remains in creative-expressive ways.[10]

Needs are physiological as well as psychological. Needs for food, drink, rest, sleep are often more imperative than needs for prestige, power, participation with others. They may be classified as primary or physiological needs, such as tissue needs for fluids, and secondary or ego needs. Each organism strives in its own way to reduce the tension generated by needs. *Man is an organism that lives in an unstable equilibrium (i.e.,* physiological, psychological, and social fluidity) *and life is the process of striving in the direction of stable equilibrium, i.e., a fixed pattern that is never reached except in death.* "Underactivity," as it has been described in other nursing literature, is a pattern in which striving or struggling is greatly inhibited, usually for psychological reasons. "Overactivity" is a pattern in which overcompensating struggle takes place. Both patterns are ways of meeting needs that are unrecognized and unmet in the present situation. Both pat-

---

[9] Iago Galdston, "On the Etiology of Depersonalization," *Journal of Nervous and Mental Diseases*, 105:25-39 (January, 1947). Suggests that when infantile satisfactions are not realized in the adult framework depersonalization results; the explanation lies in the dynamics of personalization, or ego-formation.

[10] Ralph Linton, *The Cultural Background of Personality* (New York, Appleton-Century-Crofts, Inc., 1945). See particularly chapters on "Personality" and "The Role of Culture in Personality Formation"; these two chapters elaborate a theory of motivation based on needs, particularly the need for "emotional response from other individuals."

terns of behavior are ways of using the energy generated by unmet needs.

When needs are not met in direct ways, with subsequent lowering of tension, somatic responses of greater intensity than is usual are activated. (See Fig. 16, p. 296.) These responses, being more closely related to emotional and psychological needs than to structural difficulties in the organism itself, are usually called psychosomatic responses. They require methods of study that interrelate psychological and physiological methods of inquiry; psychosomatic method is a basic one in general nursing.

Physiological changes in the body may reactivate feelings about parts of the body or the body as a whole and bring about changes in the "body image"; psychological changes in the individual may induce physiological problems and eventually lead to structural changes.

Nursing is a process that aids patients to meet their present needs so that more mature ones can emerge and be met. It is useful to observe how nurses and patients find release from tensions generated by needs and to speculate on what those needs might be. Useful transformations of energy occur when effort is directed toward recognizing together the needs of nurse and patient that have emerged in the situation and toward developing ways for achievment of satisfaction. Referring back to the summary of needs presented earlier, it can be seen that in the second one as the nurse permitted expression of needs felt by the patient—all of which were directed against others and served to disunite him from them —the patient was able to express a need pointed toward interest in developing a relationship with her. As this need is met and satisfied in the nurse-patient relationship the patient may express a need to show positive concern for members of his family. Thus, whatever need is uppermost in a hierarchy must be spent before lowermost ones, which may be more in line with health goals, can be put into service in the interest of recovery and personality development. The summary of needs in the second experience can be thought of as a repertoire of needs, all of which are ready to initiate behavior in the direction of security. The last one suggests a personal wish, a movement for something, a striving for satisfaction.

Summary

Human needs are expressed in behavior that has as its goal security or satisfaction of wants, desires, and wishes. When the work of students of the problems involved in human needs is consulted professional attitudes toward all needs expressed by patients can be designed. In general, the principle that *when needs are met new and more mature ones emerge* demands nursing skill as well as time for coming to know patients as persons. Only the patient knows what his needs are and he is not always able to identify them, knowing only that he feels the tension that needs generate. Paying attention to the needs of patients, so that personalities can develop further, is a way of using nursing as a "social force" that aids people to identify what they want and to feel free and able to struggle with others toward goals that bring satisfaction and move civilization forward. Progressive identification of needs takes place as nurse and patient communicate with one another in the interpersonal relationship.

CHAPTER 5

Interferences to Achievement of Goals

Overview

WHEN OBSTACLES stand in the way of achievement of a goal *frustration* is experienced by the patient. Nurses who recognize and appreciate those aspects of experience that are felt as frustrating to a patient and who recognize the kinds of behavior that arise in response to such experiences are in a better position to plan with the patient novel ways of meeting the difficulty. In this chapter an hypothesis on the nature and consequences of frustration will be discussed. Frustrations are common occurrences in nursing situations, as they are in all other experiences in which people are involved.

Essential questions

Every nurse has at some time said, "If I ever felt angry about anything, I certainly did this morning." It is helpful to be aware of operations that are involved in such experiences. What is it in a situation that makes one feel angry? Under what conditions do patients feel angry? How do patients express their anger? Are nurses allowed to express anger directly toward a patient? Each nurse might ask herself, "How do I respond in a situation in which I meet obstacles that impede my idea of progress?" Is my pattern of response always the same, or do I respond differently to different kinds of obstacles in different situations? What effect is my response likely to have upon me? Upon the patient? Upon my co-workers? These questions lead to critical inquiry into what is known about behavior in situations that are felt as frustrating. Discussion leads nurses to develop new attitudes toward themselves and others. A number of principles can be stated that are relevant to recurring problems in nursing situations.

Discussion

All human behavior is purposeful and goal seeking in terms of feelings of satisfaction and/or security. The purposes of human acts are not always clear; they are not always expressed in creative ways. Activity directed toward a goal is sometimes governed by forces that operate outside the awareness of an individual; unknown forces push and pull individuals in directions they do not understand. Purposes and goals are often interpreted by patients themselves, or by professional workers, as being other than that manifested in overt behavior. Professional persons may see in behavior clues or evidence about the patient to which he does not have access. Patients protest intentions that are not indicated in their acts; sometimes nurses are unaware of the discrepancy between what they say and what they do. It is not a simple matter to determine what purposes and goals direct behavior. Nurses can speculate and eventually expand their insights into human behavior.

Any interference with, blocking of, or barrier to a need, drive, or desired goal before satisfaction of these urges has been felt constitutes a frustration. Since satisfaction of needs and feeling safe and secure are outcomes of accomplishing a goal—and are therefore essential for further development of personality—a frustration often constitutes a threat to or deprivation of personality.

Dollard, Doob, *et al.*, have postulated the hypothesis that any interference with an activity started toward a goal before the responses connected with achievement of that goal are felt leads to aggression.[1] Maslow and Mittleman assert that the obstacle is frustrating when it is *perceived* as a threat to personality.[2] In order to feel frustrated there must be anticipation of a goal; an end-view, is the motivation to action as well as the purposeful aspect of activity around which personality is unified during a particular experience. Since the motivation, or stimulus, or goal, sets off and/or transforms the tension of needs or drives into energy, any interference before the energy is actually expended is perceived by the self as a barrier to action.

Application of these principles in understanding nursing situations, so that what happens can be understood, implies the necessity of looking at behavior. An observer can speculate on what are the goals, what activities toward them have been started, and what interferences or barriers to goals can be identified. Generalizations can then be made about different kinds of goals, barriers, and activities. A nurse documents a situation that illustrates these points:

Behavior observed:	*Comments and speculations:*
Recently I was asked to prepare a short talk for a staff education meeting. I tried to refuse but the supervisor was curt and pointed out that I didn't have to do it but refusal would be taken as a sign of disinterest.	An "authority figure" sets goals. The supervisor's aspirations are proposed as goals for another nurse.

[1] John Dollard, L. W. Doob, N. E. Miller, O. H. Mowrer, and R. R. Sears, *Frustration and Aggression* (New Haven, Connecticut, Yale University Press, 1939).

[2] A. H. Maslow and Bela Mittleman, *Principles of Abnormal Psychology* (New York, Harper & Brothers, 1941), p. 109.

Behavior observed:

Comments and speculations:

I reconsidered and accepted.

Accepts suggested goals.

I found that I had to spend a lot of time in preparation. Soon I became interested so that by the time of the meeting I was looking forward to making the presentation.

Activity toward the goal is started. The materials and subject generate a personal goal. How high the goal is set is not indicated, *i.e.,* her feelings are not revealed fully.

The meeting, however, was poorly conducted so that there was no time left for me to have my little say. Our time was limited so my topic was shelved indefinitely. My reaction was one of mixed feelings of disappointment, annoyance, and anger. They were directed not only toward my supervisor but my talkative co-workers as well.

An "authority figure" limits or blocks achievement of the goals set by the supervisor's suggestion and personal interest. These act as barriers.

Aggression is felt.
Diffuse, direct aggression.

She tried to apologize but I attempted to cover up my true feelings by telling her that I was glad that time ran out anyway.

Conventional attitudes operate so that she cannot communicate her real feelings to the supervisor directly.

We can see in this experience that goals were set in accordance with a need to feel secure, a need to communicate interest in the staff education program that was not felt at the time the request for active participation was made. However, as identification with the "leader's" goals became stronger, and the subject matter itself began to interest the nurse, the goal became a more personal one. Time and other nurses' talking too long were the barriers to achievement of the goal in this instance, and the aggression was partly directed toward the individuals who erected those barriers.

A second illustration serves to show a number of barriers to the achievement of a goal:[3]

Behavior observed:

As a public health nurse assigned to relieve in an area ordinarily

[3] See also discussion of this experience on p. 46.

Behavior observed:	*Comments and speculations:*
covered by another nurse, I was assigned to visit a young girl who had had contact with venereal disease. She had failed to contact the physician and co-operate in treatment.	The goal: to carry out this assignment satisfactorily.
I started out to visit the farm where the girl was living to enlist the girl's co-operation in treatment.	Activity toward the goal is started.
After making the final turn on a dirt road, I met a bull, whose lowered head made up my mind and I turned around for help. A farmer came and got the animal out of the way.	Interference #1. (Note that aggression is directed toward overcoming the difficulty, with help.)
I proceeded on my way and on reaching the farm I encountered an extremely irate mother, who felt that someone was trying to ruin her daughter's reputation.	Barrier #2. —aggression from the mother —the mother's goal to protect her daughter's reputation.
At first I was not sure that she did not have a weapon in her hand.	Aggression cannot be expressed directly; tension mounts toward anxiety; expressed as suspicion (which in this situation may have been self-protective).
I listened.	
Gradually I turned the conversation to farming and the difficulties of haying. I mentioned my episode with the bull.	Aggression is directed toward struggling through the barriers and establishing communication.
After she became quiet I explained, "No one was trying to ruin your daughter but a check to be sure that she is all right means just one trip to the doctor for examination." When I contacted the physician later he said that both mother and daughter had been in to see him.	A degree of rapport is gained and knowledge is communicated.
	Goal accomplished.

In this experience the goal of satisfaction was clearly visualized but several interferences impeded progress toward it. Barriers were easily defined and aggression that was felt was directed toward overcoming them, without varying the goal.

The relationship developed to a point where knowledge could be communicated and later acted upon, thus permitting full satisfaction to be felt by the nurse.

There are many interfering agents or obstacles that can be identified, such as conflicting habits or values leading to guilt, and the perception of personal inadequacy. (See Fig. 7, p. 95.) Disease, illness, physiological dysfunctioning are all felt as barriers to goals. Obstacles, such as the proverbial locked door, most people are familiar with. Obstacles have been classified according to their external nature; these may be active or passive, animate or inanimate, personal or impersonal. There are also obstacles of an internal nature such as psychic conflicts, as when the goal is perceived and at the same time a threat of punishment is anticipated, thus inhibiting activity toward the goal.[4] Similarly, a goal may be anticipated and interferences may occur in the form of inferior feelings perceived as "Oh, I can't do that, I'm not good enough." Inferiority as interference is a more passive internal obstacle than are threats of bodily harm, as in anticipated punishment. The nurse's goals may function as a barrier to the patient's achievement of goals toward which he is oriented.

Frustrations are related to levels of aspiration that individuals set for themselves.[5] Lewin has pointed out three factors connected with aspirations: people tend (1) to seek success, (2) to avoid failure, (3) to set goals as high as they feel they can reach and to vary them in terms of actual experiences. He has stated experimentally established facts that show: (1) The level of aspiration sought is usually high; (2) it goes up to certain points only; (3) individuals avoid areas that are too easy or too difficult.[6]

Maslow and Mittleman have shown that society can be

[4] See for example J. M. Nielson and George N. Thompson, "Schizophrenic Syndromes as Frustration Reactions," *American Journal Psychiatry*, Vol. 104, No. 12 (June, 1948), pp. 771-77.

[5] Hunt, *op. cit.*, pp. 333-78.

[6] *Ibid.*, p. 364.

frustrating, for example, in its patterns of infant care, such as clock feeding; situations set limits and raise barriers to goals; or internal factors may operate so that an individual who has an urge and an opportunity to gratify it cannot do so for psychological reasons.[7]

In studying behavior in nursing situations and attempting to discover what gives rise to aggressive behavior it is necessary to infer what motivation, drives, needs, or goals are involved and what level of aspiration is held in mind. Are the goals in line with what can be achieved within the limits of opportunity, capacity, possibility? Needs for prestige, self-esteem, and self-enhancement are often thwarted by nurse or patient in nursing situations. An illustration shows how this may operate without sufficient evidence to identify what goals are held by a patient:

Behavior observed:	*Comments and speculations:*
Mrs. X, who suffered a terminal carcinoma, was readmitted to the hospital. Her entrance created much commotion since the patient made many demands. Nurse Y, knowing the patient from a previous admission, decided to be most kind but very definite in carrying out treatments on schedule. However, this proved to be quite impossible as Mrs. X always had something important that had to be done at treatment time.	Aggressive behavior. What goals might be involved? A prior experience raises barriers and/or defines goals for the nurse. A goal is set by the nurse. The patient's immediate goals interfere with the nurse's goal.
If the nurse insisted, Mrs. X flew into a rage, shouting and screaming.	Insisting—as a way of showing aggression that cannot be shown in any other way. The imperativeness of the patient's goals is indicated in the degree of aggression that is expressed when goals cannot be reached.

[7] Maslow, *op. cit.*, pp. 113-14.

Comments and speculations:
Goals might be: the need to be
respected, to be liked, to be shel-
tered in the face of continuing
difficulty despite many hospitali-
zations. Nursing aids in the reali-
zation of these goals first.

Aggression is often related to how the nurse views the
patient and how the patient views the nurse. A child experiencing obstacles to his activities will unleash his aggression
directly, against whatever or whoever is thought to be the
aggressor. In adults, such direct expression is unacceptable
and convention dictates that aggressive feelings will be hidden. Aggression in adults is more often inhibited, redirected,
or repressed.

Aggression may be direct or indirect in its expression. (1)
When the object or person perceived to be the frustrating
source can be readily identified and aggression is directed
against that source it can be referred to as *direct aggression.*
(2) Aggression is expressed in progressively less direct manner
toward obstacles or frustrating sources that merely resemble
the original one. (That is, the nurse who reminds the patient of his wife, who raises barriers to his goals, is likely
not to get the full vent of his aggression as would his wife.)
(3) As the resemblance goes down the aggression becomes less
intense. (This may account for the fact that some nurses get
more aggression than others, due to the "resemblance cues"
they provide for the patient, although the additional factor
of permissiveness needs to be considered.) (4) When the
threat of punishment is great the possibility of indirect
aggression—toward others and toward the self—is likely.
(Hence nurses who threaten patients, by their attitudes if
not by what they say, may never experience aggression directed toward them even when they raise barriers to patient
goals.)

When frustrations are perceived repeatedly and lead to
perception of failure to accomplish goals, anxiety is experi-

enced. Anxiety, being a degree of tension that is hardly bearable, as well as a threat to personality that requires the self to defend itself in some way, demands some sort of response. Three possible responses to repeated frustrations can occur: (1) In order to achieve feelings of satisfaction the goal may be varied to one more compatible with success. Varying levels of aspiration to a goal in line with capacities, opportunities, or what is possible means taking experience into account in changing the goal. Every paraplegic patient discovers this principle. In formulating new goals, the paraplegic patient must take into account the experience in which motor and reproductive functions have been destroyed; he must identify future goals in the light of remaining capacities and opportunities. Nursing aids the paraplegic patient to take these realistic steps. (2) The response to the goal may be given up; satisfaction or security, aggression and feelings associated with it, may be dissociated. Nurses have observed many patients where the goal of recovery is given up and security is achieved through a new goal, namely, dependence upon continuing care in an institution. (3) Fixed responses may develop. These include stereotypes, delusions, fixed ideas, etc. A delusional system may develop, as in paranoia, where the goal cannot be given up or lowered and where feelings of security cannot be repressed, due to the great ego need. Fixed responses do not occur with simple frustrations; there is always an anxiety pattern of long standing that accompanies repeated frustrations that require reorganization of personality along pathological lines as relief from feelings of insecurity. An example of the development of stereotypes and its relationship to prejudice, follows:

A five-year-old child was riding on a bus with an adult. Two Negro women were also riding in the bus. In a very loud tone the child commented, "I hate those two black women over there." The adult was embarrassed and feared criticism for developing prejudices in the child, but did not moralize; instead she asked the child open-ended questions to clarify the basis for the expressed hatred. It turned out that this particular child, who seemed to have great interest in matching colors, was greatly annoyed by the fact that both women were wearing black dresses. She said, "Black people shouldn't wear black. Black doesn't go good with black. They have pretty faces and they should wear orange, or blue, or green, or some other color but not black or brown."

Then the adult commented, "Oh, you don't like the color of their dresses."

To this the child replied, "Oh, the people are all right, but they sure don't know anything about the colors that go good with them."

It is pretty well established in Social Science literature that children hate first and then accept cultural stereotypes as rationalizations in defense of their hatred or guilt for it, when it is not allowed. In other words, this child could have felt frustration if her feeling of hatred was not allowed expression and clarified; the interfering agent to her goal of expressing her feelings to her satisfaction would have been some moralizing injunction, such as, "but you mustn't hate Negroes, that is naughty." Prejudices are fixed responses that develop when feelings are cut off from expression and when prejudicial attitudes in adults in the culture are accepted as fixed responses, as an approved way of functioning in a particular locale.

The intensity of the frustration is also related to the "frustration tolerance" of an individual. Maslow and Mittleman summarize this concept of Rosenzweig as follows: Some individuals can undergo frustration without being hurt by it. What is frustrating to one individual may not be for someone else, even though they seem to be equally deprived. This factor may be related to the degree to which needs have been meet in earlier experiences. Three interacting factors seem to determine the effects of frustration: (1) the degree, (2) the need that is not met, (3) the personality of the individual in the situation.[8]

[8] Maslow, *op. cit.*, p. 115. See also S. Rosenzweig, "Frustration as an Experimental Problem," *Character and Personality*, 7:126-28 (December, 1938).

When illness is experienced as a barrier to a goal there may be three general ways in which patients react: (1) They may become more dependent than has been their pattern in adult life. (2) They may overcompensate for feelings of dependency by acting as if their independence of others was greater than that shown in previous patterns of behavior. (3)

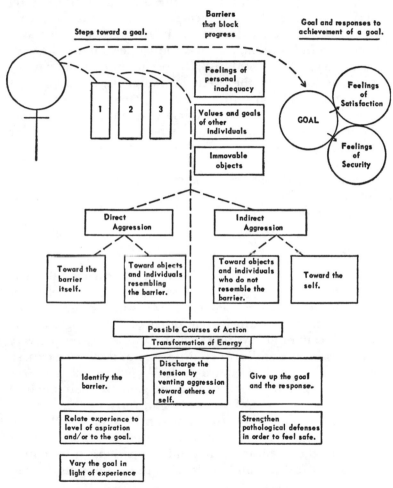

Fig. 7.   Actions involved in frustration.

They may deny the illness, acting as if the event was not being experienced. All three of these ways, it may be seen, represent responses to frustration. (1) The goal or part of the social goal—adult participation in community life—is given up in order to accept needed help during illness. (2) The goal is not given up but efforts are redoubled as a way of maintaining the illusion that the older goal and the response to it can still be reached in the new situation—continuing to work, for example (as in the patient who wants a telephone in his room, business conferences, and visits with his secretary). (3) A fixed response occurs in that the patient denies admittance of the event in awareness, dissociating it from the self and continuing to accept care and attention as if these were in the normal course of events. For example, the euphoria sometimes seen in dying patients comes under this category. The phenomenon of direct or indirect denial of illness is by no means limited to dying patients; it can be observed in multiple sclerosis, chronic disabling arthritis, amputation of limbs, and in some degree in some patients regardless of diagnosis.[9]

Summary

Frustrations are felt by everyone at some time. Barriers or interferences to goals give rise to aggressive behavior. Aggression can be direct, against the frustrating agent or obstacle, or indirect, against some other object or against the self. Goals cannot always be reached. Ordinarily, people vary their goals in line with success or failure as they have experienced them in striving toward goals. When patients set goals that are beyond what is possible, in view of their medical problem or the limits of the situation, nurses can aid them to vary the goal in line with what can be achieved. Permitting the patient to express aggression directly toward a nurse who listens therapeutically may aid the patient in becoming aware of his feelings and goals. Consistent nonpunitiveness

[9] See example, pp. 66-67.

and a nonjudgmental attitude toward the patient's aggression may make it possible for the patient to reflect upon and to doubt the validity of his present behavior, as well as the need for it in relating to a mature nurse who accepts him as he is. Threats of punishment that are perceived in the situation or that function as internal barriers often lead to indirect expression of aggression. Patients who are self-punishing may injure themselves physically. Nursing goals are often obstacles to the patient's goals; communication in the interpersonal relationship aids both the nurse and the patient to clarify their goals and to reach common understanding.

CHAPTER **6**

Opposing Goals

Overview

IN ALL SITUATIONS in which nursing is practiced, whatever interaction between nurse and patient is observed can be examined and studied in the light of the basic principle that the direction of human behavior is forward. Regression is a concept that is well accepted in psychiatry but nurses can speculate on its validity; it is possible that an individual learns about living with people in relation to specific tools available at various eras of development and in relation to specific tasks that require learning in these eras.[1] It is further possible that individuals build a conventional superstructure of accomplishments upon the base line in terms of actual learning, and that when this superstructure no longer works, earlier capacities or tools are again put to use, and the point at which learning to live with people has stopped or the base line of actual learning can be identified. Then it can be seen that the basic direction is forward, that there is a continuing attempt to complete a task in learning at a specific era, which may have long been passed in terms of chronological age. Keener observation in clinical situations will clarify the hypotheses that the basic direction is forward and that what is meant by regression is the use of earlier capacities in relation to earlier unmet tasks. These

[1] See Part III.

unmet tasks were sufficiently covered up so that it looked as though subsequent learning about living with people had taken place until a crisis situation occurred.

It is sometimes difficult to understand that behavior is goal directed in situations where goals are interfered with and aggression is expressed. The situation becomes more complex and more difficult to understand when behavior, as it is expressed in an interpersonal situation, involves two opposing goals. The purpose of this chapter is to identify principles that operate when an individual is undergoing conflict, to understand behavior that is influenced by two opposing goals competing for dominance. Conflict of some kind and in some degree is always present in individuals or in their culture. It is inevitable in the process of living. In this culture, conflict between the values of an industrial society and the values reflected in humanistic thought are examples of opposites that are difficult to reconcile. American boys and girls are expected to compete successfully with others, to strive for prestige and status beyond that of their parents, and to prepare themselves for a future that includes an increasing salary as they grow older. On the other hand, they are taught to love one another, to be concerned about the affairs of their neighbor, and to give no thought to storing up material possessions in this world. Each boy and girl grapples with these opposing value systems. Each patient is caught in conflicts of competing value systems.

A discussion of conflict, and the behavior that ensues when it is present, can profitably be centered around principles that govern responses to conflict and methods individuals use for developing awareness of and resolution of conflicts.

Essential questions

How can two goals held by the same individual direct behavior? What kinds of behavior indicate the presence of conflict? How do people feel when they undergo conflict? If conflict has to do with opposing goals, I wonder if that is why I get a headache when I have to do things that the supervisor tells me to do but that I feel I should not do? What do I need to know about conflict in order to help myself and others? Is it necessary for nurses to pay attention to conflicts that patients feel; isn't that the job of a psychiatrist?

Possible generalizations are suggested by experiences nurses have had. Two experiences are cited.

Nurse:

One day I was sitting on a bench in the park reading an assignment. On the bench next to mine there sat a very attractive young lady. My attention was directed to her because, for about an hour, she seemed oblivious to her environment. Finally, she turned her head and our eyes met. She seemed to stare at me for a moment, as though she recognized me, then abruptly arose and came to where I was sitting. She looked like a sleepwalker; she was neatly and expensively dressed in a blue ensemble. Without further ado she sat down and talked while I listened.

(Note that the nurse has not said anything. Note, too, the strength of mother disapproval in the girl's present standards of behavior.)

(Note how the mother's standards operate to determine what she can do.)

(The nurse makes no comment; none is expected.)

Stranger in the park:

What are you reading?
I came down here to watch the boats. I quit my job yesterday. It was a pretty good job but I am going away. I wish I could go home, but I can't because my mother thinks I'm a failure. I never could get myself a suitable husband like my sister. Oh, I could have married lots of boys at home but they were so provincial—no money, you see, and mother thinks money is awfully important.
Do you like New York? I hate it. I've been here a year and I haven't a single friend. Everyone is so

Nurse:

(Others are not evaluated on the basis of how they relate to her but where they came from.)

(The theme—you can get used to the things you are afraid of; this is different from coming to know them.)

(Note the feelings projected onto the apartment.)

(Note the self-punitive indirect aggression to barriers set by mother's goal for her.)

(Uncritical acceptance and strengthening of goal of mother —money—and vague suggestion of a personal goal.)

(Indecision is identified by her. Note that crying is a tool useful in infancy.)

Who is Joan?

(The first comment by the nurse.)

(Note how appraisals that the mother has made of men operate in the responses she makes.)

(Note the conflict between marriage and career.)

Would you tell me your name and where you live?

Stranger in the park:

standoffish and I feel I can never trust them; you never know where they live, or who their families are. I'm going to Japan. That's why I came here to watch the boats. I'm afraid of boats and I want to get used to the look of a boat because I'll have to be on one for a long time.

I just couldn't stay in the apartment any more; it is so impersonal and lonesome. Today I decided to jump out of the window, then maybe mother would realize how hard it was for me to be a success on her terms. I've got my things all packed and I'm going to New Jersey at five o'clock. At least I think I am if Joan doesn't forget. She doesn't want me to go to Japan but I got a job there and I'll be able to save lots of money. Everything is cheap in Japan. I'm a good secretary and I know I will be a success there.

Oh dear, I am so upset, I don't know what to do. (At this point she started to cry, then stared out toward the river.)

Oh, Joan is the only friend I have, but she is married—to the right kind of husband, too. Mother would approve of him; he has a flare for always doing the right thing and looking always like a collar ad. Last night I called Joan just to talk to her. She told me to pack my things and be here today at five o'clock. She'll probably forget to come; she's so busy being happy with her husband. (Crying again.)

Nurse:

(Up to this point the nurse has remained an anonymous sounding board against which she could reveal her feelings; note the arousal of anxiety when the nurse asked her to reveal who she is. The nurse felt anxious about the stranger and communicated it.) It's four-thirty. You will have twenty minutes before Joan will be here. Would you like me to walk along home with you to see if she has arrived. I really need the exercise.

Stranger in the park:

Oh, forgive me, I'm terribly sorry to have bothered you with all this, but it has been wonderful talking to you. I guess I'll have to be going. What time is it?

But you don't know me at all. I don't know why you should bother about me, no one else ever does. But if you would like to come, I'd like you to. I'm afraid of that horrible apartment. I just can't stand it anymore. Gosh, I don't know what I will do if Joan doesn't come. I wish I could go home, but I can't go. I just can't and have mother ask me again why I can't get myself a decent husband.

The evidence given is not sufficient to identify exactly what two goals are opposed in the present conflict. We can speculate that there is a need to feel close to others, to be able to count on them for fulfilling wishes connected with dependence. The girl's dependence upon Joan, permitting the nurse to walk home with her are movements toward people who will help. However, a stronger goal seems to be that of avoiding dependence upon her mother, which might be expected if she were to go home. Although she responds, uncritically, in terms of goals she attributes to her mother, her expectations are not that these goals will be fulfilled but that they will be avoided by going to some faraway land. While she approaches Joan and the nurse, seeking help of some kind, more effort is exerted in planning a way to avoid going home. Earlier unmet needs for dependence probably require submission to her mother's wishes. These speculations might lead to further understanding of the behavior expressed in this situation when more evidence is available.

An experience in a surgical ward provides another opportunity to make generalizations from everyday experience, which can later be verified or disproved in other situations.

Mrs. Jones was the mother of two girls, ages seven and nine. She came to the hospital for a mastectomy. Immediately after the operation "she behaved in the usual manner of trying to accept and adapt to the situation." In a few days she seemed fairly comfortable; she was relieved that the operation was over and expressed eagerness to go home. She expressed the wish to take care of her children and the possibility that they were being neglected.

So far, the case materials show what might be two opposing goals: to remain in the hospital situation and complete the experience that she was undergoing, taking care of herself and understanding the event; a second goal seems to be that of going home and forgetting the surgical experience as she takes care of others in her role of mother. The case material continues:

After about a week her attitudes changed. She expressed many reasons why she could not go home. She felt there was no solution to her problems. She would look grotesque in her clothes and might not be able to go swimming. The children would notice that she was disfigured. In all discussion with the nurse she shifted from one goal to the other: she wanted to go home but she couldn't.

Deeper underlying goals motivate the behavior described in this case material. But as the nurse faces this recurring problem, with many patients from different socioeconomic backgrounds, the issues as stated are the ones she faces—not the underlying psychic conflicts. The nurse can help the patient when she appreciates the meaning of the action in the drama unfolding in her relations with the patient. Several principles help to clarify what is happening.

Conflict, like frustration, is a compelling experience that increases tension and thus provides energy as a crucial factor in behavior. According to experimental studies in conflict, as summarized by Miller, conflict forces a choice that is often expressed in behavior that seems to others to be inappropriate for the situation.[2] Shifting from one goal to another, searching out reasons why one can and yet cannot go home, distracts and delays attention to the deeper difficulty—the conflict in feelings that are held about the two possibilities. Such distractions ultimately fatigue the patient so that alertness is reduced. Factors that would illuminate the difficulty are not so likely to be taken into account and an intelligent choice becomes more difficult to make. Liddell's work, in experimentally created conflicts in animals, has provided certain evidence: When conflict is created by a situation, or by expected responses to it, the animal is unable to make the necessary discriminations. Hence, a maladaptive response resolves the conflict.[3]

Miller, who bases his hypotheses on experimental studies refers to responses such as *hesitation, tension, vacillation, or complete blocking* as ones that are produced when there is competition between incompatible responses to drives.[4] However, not all competition between incompatible responses gives rise to hesitancy. Every situation calls out many responses in an individual. There is an order to the way responses are made. A dominant one is made first, then a next dominant one follows, until all responses required have been made. In conflict, however, a stalemate is reached only when there is complete blocking; responses in the direction of approaching a goal and other ones aimed at avoiding another goal incompatible with the first one lead to "stable equilibrium." Miller identifies four principles to account for the stalemate. These principles are restated here:

1. As the subject comes closer to the goal his tendency to approach it becomes stronger.

[2] J. McV. Hunt (ed.), *Personality and the Behavior Disorders* (New York, The Ronald Press Company, 1944), Vol. I, pp. 431-465.
[3] Hunt, *op. cit.,* pp. 389-413.
[4] *Ibid.,* pp. 431-65.

2. As the subject comes closer to a goal to be avoided his tendency to avoid it becomes stronger.
3. As the subject comes nearer to the goal the tendency to avoid a goal rapidly increases its strength; this rapid strengthening of the tendency is *not* noticed in the tendency to approach a goal.
4. The strength of each drive or goal changes the strength of approach and avoidance and this may change the outcome.

Conflict can be said to be present only when tendencies for avoidance are present. For example, when the patient says that he doesn't want to stay in the hospital, and is eager to go home, but doesn't act eager, reasons for avoidance can be speculated on. According to the principles just cited, the drives to stay and to go home being equal, the tendency to avoid going home would in all probability become stronger as the date of discharge from the hospital draws near. However, for the patient who actually has a strong wish or drive to go home but a less strong desire to remain, the approach drive would gain ascendancy and this goal would materialize without the patient showing vacillating behavior. It is helpful to keep in mind that when the tendency to approach and to avoid are both relatively strong tendencies the oscillation produced will be more noticeable; the patient will have greater difficulty in reaching a decision on what to do. It can be repeated that the drives and goals that underlie the behavior seen in clinical situations are often different from ones cited as "going home" or "not going home." These are the ways that nurses face the difficulty with the patient.

Miller points out that there are many types of incompatibility of responses that lead to conflict behavior. These include:[5]

1. Mechanical—motor incompatibility based upon physical structure.

[5] *Ibid.*, pp. 456-59.

2. Neural—for example, the failure of reciprocal innervation in muscular functioning.

3. Chemical—such as the adrenalin secreted when fear is experienced, which improves functioning in relation to avoidance of the feared object but interferes with digestive functioning.

4. Perceptual—when a child hears a voice but the person speaking cannot be seen.

5. Acquired—for example, conflicting feelings of love and hatred toward the same person; ideas that are logically contradictory when applied to a problem; contrasting expressions of feelings.

Miller points out and seems to verify in his experiments Freud's earlier contention that withdrawal or fear are signs that strong tendencies to approach are present. It is a valuable lead for nurses that withdrawal behavior in itself indicates that equally strong approach behavior may be present. The issue then becomes one of *how the professional persons in the situation can release in patients the tendencies to identify and to approach a goal.* However, a patient showing deep withdrawal seems to verify another principle, namely, that conflicts solved by avoidance tend to generalize to more and more areas of life and thus tend to make all choices more difficult. This appears evident in the first experience cited in this chapter, *i.e.,* of the stranger in the park.[6]

A relationship between fear and conflict can be recognized. When fear is the source of avoidance, the feared object can be identified and thus avoided; from the educative standpoint the feared object may be explored and become known, thus reducing the strength of avoidance. Thus, the patient who fears having a basal metabolism is permitted to see the apparatus, have an explanation of how it works and what is expected of him, and perhaps even a trial run to reduce the strength of avoidance. However, when unexplained anxiety

6 See pp. 101-103.

is present, it is necessary to look for internal conflicts.[7] A patient who states that he fears an object may be using that object as a way of focalizing more deeply felt concerns; the object may symbolize or stand for an event that has greater meaning to him than is apparent in behavior; therefore, the nurse may be helping the patient in a situation in which internal conflicts arise but are not verbalized.[8]

Horney speaks of normal conflict as the making of choices between goals both of which are desirable.[9] Miller would refer to this as approach-approach competition.[10] However, Horney identifies "neurotic conflicts" as ones in which choice is impossible for the individual; he is carried along in making decisions by underlying desires that are not known to him and that have a compulsive quality to them.[11] Many students of the problems involved in conflict assert that the two drives are incompatible, contradictory, irreconcilable. Lewin has shown why approach-approach competition, leading to unstable equilibrium fails to produce behavior seen in conflict, such as indecision, vacillation, blocking.[12] The essential difference between situations in which avoidance operates and those in which both goals can be approached lies in their effect upon equilibrium.

In the chapter on Human Needs (Chapter 4), it has been pointed out that satisfaction of wants and the need to feel safe or secure are two main directive goals influencing behavior. In the two examples introduced in this chapter it can be seen that the wants, or wishes, of the individuals relating to the nurses were not clear. Both knew what they did not want. Both oriented their behavior in terms of avoiding what they did not want, in order to feel safe and secure.

[7] Hunt, *op. cit.,* p. 451.

[8] See Chapter 12, Communication.

[9] Karen Horney, *Our Inner Conflict* (New York, W. W. Norton & Company, 1945), p. 32.

[10] Hunt, *op. cit.,* p. 432.

[11] Horney, *op. cit.,* p. 32.

[12] C. Murchinson, *A Handbook of Child Psychology* (Worcester, Massachusetts, Clark University Press, 1931), paper by Kurt Lewin, "Environmental Forces in Child Behavior and Development."

Both were inattending, or denying entrance into awareness, their feelings connected with goals that they might want. Neither the wants nor goals, nor the feelings connected with them, emerged very clearly. Many feelings connected with what they were against were expressed. In both individuals these feelings were also connected with the way they felt about themselves and what others might think about them.

In the two situations discussed the nurses permitted expression of feelings without interposing ones that were judgmental or that suggested how the individuals in question "should" feel. That is, they provided full exploration of dominant feelings as a way of attempting to reduce the strength of avoidance. It is to be noted that when the nurse asked the young girl in the park the question, "Who are you?" with all that may have been perceived to be inherent in the question, the young girl became defensive. That is, *she felt threatened and defended herself by strengthening her tendency to avoid relations with people.* When the nurse did not press the question, but reinforced the interest that the stranger must have felt, the girl was able to move toward her. That is, her tendency to approach people, even though on a basis of dependence, was slightly strengthened. We do not know what might have been the outcome over a long period of time, nor whether both nurses could have sustained their helpfulness through all that would be required in these relationships, but the evidence does show what was happening at the time it was gathered.

The task in nursing situations, where patients experience conflicting goals, and all of the discomfort in making choices that they may or may not be able to make wisely, is to *listen.* The nurse's acting as a sounding board against which the patient can ventilate and recognize what he feels permits the patient to become aware of the evidence on which a choice can be made. Interpretation of the meaning of what is said and felt is often perceived as a barrier to the goal of talking it out, namely, becoming aware of what is felt. As has already been pointed out in the chapter on frustration (Chapter 5) aggression can be expected when a goal or its activity is interfered with. In conflict situations, where the feelings connected with one of the goals, usually the goal to be avoided, are interfered with, aggression is most frequently expressed in terms of a fixed response. That is, it is difficult in a conflict situation to vary goals, or to give up goals or responses connected with them, and consequently defense dynamisms are brought into play.

Everyone uses defense dynamisms in some degree in some situations. Their function is to aid forward movement by reinforcing feelings of safety in a situation that seems threatening. The operation has been thought of as that of falling back to concentrate forces, in order to move ahead with greater feelings of personal power. In conflict, when the tendency to approach a goal is inhibited or adequately repressed, the tendency to avoid gains strength. If new conditions are provided in the situation and the avoidance is not challenged—requiring further defense of self—the individual will begin to find ways to reduce its strength and thus to move forward in noticeable ways. However, any relationship that challenges the adequacy of the repression of the approach drive, for instance, a nurse who constantly assures· the patient that she must go home and that everything will be all right there inadvertently strengthens the tendency to avoid. Comments are made to the effect, "I talked with her for hours about her readiness to go home but she seems more eager to stay now than ever before." A new condition can be introduced into the situation if the nurse comments, "You feel that you cannot go home. Perhaps we can talk about it if you wish." This kind of comment does not require the patient to push responses and feelings connected with avoidance of going home out of awareness, and thus does not strengthen the tendency to avoidance in a way that may influence spreading to other behavioral systems as conflict deepens.

A relationship that is useful to the patient is one in which what is expected of him is made clear and adhered to consistently, with regard to mechanical procedures and treatment, and one in which he is treated with understanding and respect as a person. Such respect includes the right to have his own feelings and to express them in the presence of professional persons who may understand them, but who will not necessarily confront the patient with the intention of his feelings. A psychiatrist may deem it wise to interpret difficulties directly with the patient; a nurse whose changing roles require that she shuttle between being a resource person, a surrogate, a counselor cannot make interpretations of feelings without endangering her usefulness in all of her roles.

The nurse can talk directly with the patient about how he is getting along. She can say how she feels about the patient when this seems necessary. She can aid the patient to come to know her as a person who is like all others in some ways and unique in other ways. She can listen intelligently. Where professional teams operate the nurse may seek day-by-day guidance in collaborative efforts with other professional workers in specific situations. Even with these enlightened ways of relating to patients, all of which are dependent upon the extent of functional understanding—what each nurse observes and knows at a given moment—defensive responses in patients undergoing conflict are still likely.

Defensive responses that operate and are strengthened when an individual perceives the need to avoid a goal can be seen in the two experiences cited. *Introjection,* or the incorporation into the self or ego-system of attitudes and feelings that others have shown during formative years, were seen in the young girl's use of "images" of her mother. This is a normal dynamism that young children and others use, as a way of becoming socialized. The danger in introjection, and the use of it in an extreme or pathological degree, lies in the possibility of conferring upon the image the status of an individual who walks and/or talks with and thus controls what another individual does. This was evident in the young girl's decisions and expressions of feelings—all of which reflected the governing power of an absent mother in ways that defeated her development as a person in her own right. Sometimes patients are governed by a dead parent, or wife, who seems to be present and taking an active hand in present behavior This is often markedly noticeable in individuals undergoing depression when a loved one actually dies. An individual may keep the departed one's room in order, retain all of the clothes, and seem to communicate with a figure now departed this life, rather than with persons in the present situation.

Projection is another defense dynamism that everyone uses in some degree at some time during life. Blame avoidance is common in children. Adults shift blame toward others saying, "They should give us better conditions in this city," "They should improve this situation," and the like. The noticeable lack of the operation of the self-dynamism in improving conditions or enriching situations is apparent; it is assigned to others who may or may not be identifiable in the community or the situation. Projection becomes pathological, that is, it operates in extreme degree when all problems, all difficulties, all painful ideas that actually arise in the self—at least in large part—are attributed to or blamed upon others. The young girl in the park expressed the feelings that others were "standoffish and I can never trust them," "the apartment was impersonal and lonesome"—feelings that an apartment could not have. There is not sufficient evidence to show how strong is this tendency to shift blame upon others but it is noticeable how the process of dissociating these feelings from the self and attributing them to others got started. We can speculate that this individual, as a child, was appraised in these ways by her mother, if not by others. that she was made to feel that she could not be trusted, that she was standoffish, that she was impersonal and lonesome. These feelings being intolerable ones, that make her feel unsafe, require some defense that restores a measure of security. The girl feels safer attributing her feelings and thoughts to others.

Sublimation is a third defense dynamism that operates in normal degree shading into extreme degree for many individuals. It is a process by which patterns of behavior that express primitive, or instinctual, needs or forces are replaced by ways of behaving that are more acceptable in the social milieu in which one finds oneself. In extreme degree a variety of needs and wishes are all telescoped into one form of activity that substitutes for and becomes an all-encompassing interest in the life of that individual. Many channels of sublimation are possible for an individual whose personality is flexible and open to examination; a self that cannot be examined and that perceives inquiry as a threat that demands immediate fixed responses is likely to reach one channel that appeases. The stranger in the park mentioned only her ability in her job as one in which all of her wishes and needs might find expression; even her friend Joan was not a channel fully open to her because of her own feelings about others.

Many other dynamisms operate to provide security when personality is threatened.[13] They are used when barriers are perceived as one goal is pursued; they also provide security when two incompatible goals operate and making a decision between them is impossible.

Horney points out three types of individual trends in interpersonal relations that have to do with attempts at resolution of inner conflicts.[14] These trends operate in conjunction with defenses against threats to personality, as discussed above. (1) When feelings of helplessness and of powerlessness operate an individual may show a *tendency to move*

[13] In the author's opinion an excellent source on defense dynamisms is: Percival Symonds, *Dynamics of Human Adjustment* (New York, Appleton-Century-Crofts, Inc., 1946).

[14] Horney, *op. cit.*, pp. 42-43. See also: Patrick Mullahy, *Oedipus: Myth and Complex* (New York, Hermitage House, Inc., 1949), pp. 230-31.

toward, or approach, others as a way of feeling safe. Attachment to and compliance with other individuals who are felt to be stronger is a way of decreasing feelings of weakness and at the same time a way of gaining a feeling of being attached to or belonging to others. (2) When the intentions of others are distrusted and there is need to express hostility and revenge in order to defeat others, and thus to feel personal strength, an individual may show a *tendency to move against others. This is a way of avoiding relations* with them in order to feel safe against the intrusion of what they may expect should be done. (3) When an individual feels isolated and alone and feels that he holds nothing of common interest and that others do not understand his needs, *a tendency to avoid people may be shown in moving away from them.*

Horney points out further that these three patterns most often are mixed but that one predominates and is observable in what happens in an interpersonal relationship. A fourth and more positive movement can be added, although each of the above three movements can often be viewed as a step in this direction. (4) When a wish is felt to participate actively with others in the solution of common problems and an individual feels that he is fully accepted and respected as a person who can and does make choices, *a tendency to move with others on the basis of collaborative relations is observable.* Active participation requires that others recognize that one can make a contribution to the solutions of problems that arise in daily living; more importantly, however, it requires that an individual will recognize powers within himself that make it possible for him to share his feelings, experiences, and knowledge with others.

All nursing situations can be studied in terms of operation of these four trends and can lead to participation in the solution of interpersonal problems. Horney points out repeatedly the relationship between conditions that give rise to conflicting tendencies and the therapeutic importance of providing new conditions under which the individual can "retrieve himself." The development of awareness of one's own feelings, evolving one's own set of goals and values, and relating one's self positively to others, that is, on the basis of translating one's convictions into action, are three tasks each individual faces. Interpersonal conditions that make it possible for a patient to meet these tasks and in some degree to master the difficulties involved and to develop skills required for further mastery are more likely to be provided when the nurse and patient relationship is studied.

It is customary in all of the professions to view the professional person as outside of the patient's problem—to see the patient as if he were standing over in a corner where he could be observed with complete detachment and without recourse to the situation in which the patient is behaving. To examine the evidence fully requires that the actions of the nurse, what she says, feels, thinks, does, in relation to what the patient does, become the subject of inquiry, too. The patient responds in a situation and to the people who are in it. Fruitful inquiry requires all of the evidence in order to find out what happens in a situation that reinforces tendencies to approach or to avoid or to participate with others.

Constructive resolution of conflicts that underlie behavior often requires therapy of an uncovering type.[15] This kind of therapy is offered by a psychiatrist, a psychoanalyst, or a psychiatrically oriented internist. However, a nursing relationship can help the patient to express and become aware of his feelings about present perplexities and problems. This requires recognition of tendencies that operate in the relationship, early recognition and delimitation of boundaries in the situation in which the patient acts out his feelings, professional responses to needs and wishes expressed, and acceptance of the *patient as he is*. Acceptance of a patient who is in coma, or otherwise completely helpless, is at first unconditional. The relationship of nurse to patient, however, moves on a continuum from unconditional care to participant

[15] Horney, *op. cit.*, pp. 219-20.

relations in which both can collaborate on the solution of nursing problems.[16]

Summary

Two opposing goals can operate to distort interpersonal relations and to deflect the patient from the tasks involved in planning to meet his medical problem. The goals are incompatible with each other and one or both may not be clearly visualized, the patient acting on goals that operate outside of awareness. The presence of conflict is recognized when a patient shows hesitation, vacillation, and/or blocking and inability to decide on a course of action to be followed. A tendency to avoid activities, people, exploration of personal feelings is observable. Conflict gives rise to tension which may be relieved through active inquiry into the difficulties and felt concerns of the patient. The energy that derives from tension can also become bound in symptoms, such as headache, unexplained fever, a need to put aside the problem and lose oneself in some other kind of work, or suicidal intentions or acts. Some of these symptoms were seen in the two experiences presented in this chapter. A nurse can help patients when she appreciates the actions involved and the transformation of energy that takes place. (See Fig. 7, p. 95.) The ability to approach a problem and to utilize the energy available for expression in this ability is developed when a patient is permitted to have and to express his own feelings. Nursing aids the patient to become aware of how he feels about his present predicament as a way of helping him to clarify and to act upon goals. Conflict is a common, recurring problem that is faced by all individuals in all walks of life in some degree. Conflicts expressed in the presence of nurses are often in the form of peripheral problems, to stay in the hospital or to go home, rather than in the form of deeper central conflicts, such as to be dependent or independent. Skills in

[16] Full discussion of the actions involved follows in Part III, Psychological Tasks.

meeting problems, and tendencies to avoid a problem, are re-inforced in every new situation in which an individual finds himself. By using the experience of illness as a situation in which learning takes place nursing fosters the development of skills for participation in the solution of problems.

CHAPTER 7

Unexplained Discomfort

Overview

UNEXPLAINED DISCOMFORT, such as needs, frustration, and conflict, is an experience that influences behavior by providing energy. While many of the internal (psychobiological) and external (cultural) forces that impel individuals in forward or backward movement of personality are not fully understood, much has been written about needs, frustration, and conflict, and about *anxiety*. All of these experiences act as instrumentalities in the continuing reorganization of experience and in reconstruction of personality. Such reorganization and reconstruction can be productive or nonproductive. Productive relations with others can be fostered more readily when the interaction that takes place in an interpersonal relationship and its meanings are understood. In order to make clear the demands these experiences make upon an individual and their energizing quality, these experiences have been separated into four chapters. In actual operation they occur in combination. The purpose of this chapter is to identify and to clarify the nature of anxiety, as it occurs in nurses, in patients, and its communication in the interpersonal relationship. Relations with psychological experiences already discussed will be shown. An orientation to the usefulness and the dangers involved when these psychological experiences are undergone by patients will allow a

119

more critical evaluation of the effects of interpersonal performances in nursing situations.

Essential questions

Many nurses have asserted: I can understand a patient who is uncomfortable right after an operation but these patients that complain about discomfort when the doctors can't find anything wrong puzzle me! What gives rise to such discomfort? Some patients seem to be apprehensive about nothing! Others seem to lack faith in all of us; they seem to want to be sick all the rest of their lives! Some of them act as if they are so guilty that they cannot allow us to do anything for them! Once in a while a patient is so upset that we have literally to pour sedatives into her to get her quiet! I wonder what these kinds of discomfort are all about? I wonder if I need to find out in order to help these patients? We are so busy all of the time and the patients who make so many demands, and yet don't seem to know what it is that they want, take up a lot of time needed for other work. These are everyday assertions or questions that show recognition of the relationship between the patient's discomfort and unmet demands on nursing service.

There are other problems that arise that involve knowledge of principles of anxiety, but these more often go unrecognized. Why won't John Jones eat? Mr. Smith simply must have that enema but he goes wild when I try to give it to him! A five-year-old boy who was badly burned and had to be taken to the operating room every day, for cleansing the areas and for redressing them, always had to have a preliminary hypodermic and anesthesia. Soon he became so frightened that even these worked more slowly and it was difficult to administer them. Why wouldn't this boy cooperate with us? Many problems arise every day in nursing situations that require knowledge and application of principles for the achievement of understanding and useful consequences. What are the psychological principles that illuminate what is involved in situations where patients feel anxious? This chapter outlines some of the actions and principles involved.

A nurse documents the following experience from which generalizations can be made:

Patient:

A patient, who was 6 ft. 5 in. tall and had a special seven-foot bed, employed a private duty nurse. On arrival he looked her over from head to foot and seemed disappointed. "Why did they send me such a tiny nurse? Why you are barely eighteen! When did you finish your training? Did you have any experience in taking care of a surgical patient? You know I had a big operation this morning!" (This patient was a doctor.) "I am not a fussy patient like most doctors but I want everything just right. Now I can't see how you can help me much with your size."

The patient was quiet for a while and then very often asked for the urinal, passing only two or three ounces each time. He appeared restless.
(Apprehension was expressed in frequent urination and restlessness.)

Nurse:

I could feel that he was disappointed when he saw me but I didn't know why.

I told him where and when I had finished my training and said, "I am older than you think I am." (This nurse was very tiny.)

I was irked by his picking on my size. (The nurse expressed her aggression by saying) "Of course you don't expect me to pick you up, but I can always help you to turn on your sides and help yourself. If I can't do it I can always ask the floor nurse or the orderly to help me."
(The nurse gives information on how she plans to approach the problem the patient perceives.)
"Meantime, suppose you relax and tomorrow the nursing office will get you another big nurse. Are you comfortable?"

(Was the nurse's need for prestige threatened? Did she have expectations that her needs would be met in this situation when her efforts were recognized and appreciated? Did the patient's preconceptions about nurses and the nurse's pre-

Patient:

Nurse:

conceptions about doctors operate to distort this relationship and to make both parties anxious?)

"Oh, it's just my heart. It is acting queer. Call my doctor right away. I want to see him."
(The patient decides on a course of action that will relieve his anxiety.)
(The nurse gave a medication that was ordered P.R.N. and then called the doctor.)

(Did the nurse communicate her anxiety to the patient and thus force him to rely upon the doctor who could be trusted and with whom he could feel safe?)
I called the doctor and he ordered a second hypodermic which I prepared and gave.

"Is he coming? If this is Demerol I don't want it. That crazy stuff. I want to see my doctor right now."
(The patient was insistent about seeing his doctor as his anxiety began to mount. He expressed that he was afraid to die.)

(Was the nurse *sorry* for this patient who was afraid he might die, and at the same time *irritated* because he was a doctor and should therefore "know better" than to be upset and apprehensive? Is there a conflict in feelings in this nurse?)
"Well if you refuse to be injected I will tell your doctor, shall I?"

The patient was quiet and trying hard to decide.
"Are you sure your needle is sharp and sterile? You know, such care-lessness can cause abscess, it happens many times, you know."
(The patient took the hypo.)
"Is it over? Is the needle intact? I have seen cases where nurses break needles and you know I don't want that to happen. But you have light hands."

I assured him that the needle was sharp and everything was sterile.

I gave the patient a backrub and made him comfortable. "Try to sleep now. I know that you are very tired and sleepy. I will be here all of the time."

The patient slept at long inter-vals without any further "com-plaints" until morning. "I slept well. I was sorry I was rather rude

Patient:

to you last night. But now I
think you are O.K. in spite of
your size. I am glad you are not
like other nurses who stay out of
the rooms."

In analyzing the evidence presented it can be seen that
*each party in the two-way relationship had conceptions about
what the other was like and that these preconceptions operated before they came to know one another.* Although no
specific effort was made to identify the preconceptions held
by each, what was expected was partly revealed. The patient
expected a nurse who would be larger than this tiny one,
the nurse would do everything "just right"—whatever that
means to the patient—and carry out procedures without
hurting him and stay with him in the room all night. Because he incidentally happened to be a physician, we can
assume that he had considerable opportunity in working with
nurses to develop a picture of what one who took care of
him *should* be like. Although the evidence does not show
explicitly what expectations the nurse had in mind of a
patient who was also a doctor, we can see that she expected
him to be able to manage his own feelings, that she could
speak forthrightly to him and not be intimidated by his
covert aggression aimed at destroying her self-esteem. When
the nurse met the patient's expectations he could accept her
as an individual who was like other nurses and different from
them. These expectations were relatively simple: to call his
doctor when he wished it, to make him comfortable, to stay
in the room with him during the night. The evidence does
not identify it explicitly but when the doctor met the nurse's
expectations, by sleeping well, by praising her efforts and
commenting on what pleased him, she was able to develop
a relationship and remain with him for the duration of his
illness.

The nurse might have explored her own feelings further
and helped the patient to explore his. She might have said,

"You want me to do everything right but you can't see how a tiny person like me can do it." Or, "You think I might be careless in giving this hypodermic to you as other nurses whom you know have been." These responses *do not* seal up the possibilities for identifying feelings and other sources that aid the patient to learn about himself and the way he is operating in this situation. Saying "I have never had an abscess form in any patient to whom I have given a hypodermic" is a way of defending one's own prestige that often closes off further communications beyond what is necessary for mechanical assistance.

Another generalization can be made. Looking at the evidence we can see that anxiety developed and was strengthened after the nurse entered the situation. The patient became restless, urinated more frequently in smaller amounts, and felt that his heart was "acting queer." We can see, too, that many feelings were called out in the nurse: she was irked; she threatened to tell the patient's doctor; she probably felt sorry and irritated with the patient. In general, *the anxiety arose, developed, and became more severe for both parties in this situation as they communicated their discomfort to one another.* Sullivan points out that this is the unique characteristic of anxiety: *its interpersonal induction in situations in which prestige and dignity are threatened by others from whom one cannot escape.*[1] Certainly the nurse's feelings of worth-whileness and of self-respect were threatened. The patient's need for prestige, as evidenced in the idea of nurse he had in mind—which he could not immediately escape —was also threatened. Some of these circumstances were amenable to control but not at the outset of the relationship. There isn't any way that the preconceptions of two people can be matched in advance so that anxiety will not be felt. There is the possibility that the nurse will develop *skill in aiding the patient to undergo the discomfort and to utilize*

[1] H. S. Sullivan, *The Meaning of Anxiety in Psychiatry and in Life* (Washington, D.C., William Alanson White Psychiatric Foundation, 1948) pamphlet, pp. 11-12.

the energy provided by the anxiety in identifying and assessing the difficulties in the situation. This was not done in the experience cited and accounts for the spread of anxiety in the patient, to his heart, to his urinary apparatus, and so forth. The difficulty was solved by giving two hypodermics, which aided the patient to avoid the discomfort and to avoid further recognition of his feelings about himself and about nurses. Sleep intervened and if this is the goal of the relationship it can be said that the goal has been achieved. However, if the goal is that of aiding the patient to integrate illness as an experience that has happened to him and through which he can learn more about himself than was known before, activities toward this goal would have preceded the induction of sleep. Going to sleep because the work of the day is finished and forcing oneself to sleep in order to avoid whatever work remains are two different modes of responding to difficulty.

If the reader will turn back to page 66 and review the case materials presented there, it will be noted that, when feelings are not permitted expression and identified, the genuine feelings connected with the illness as an experience are dissociated and thereafter operate outside awareness and outside of control of the individual. There are many ways to force avoidance of the problem: urging concentration on work in the future, diverting attention from feelings that are expressed to feelings that *should* be held, and by giving large quantities of sedatives, which aid the processes of forgetting.

Nursing is an interpersonal process that co-operates with and assists natural ongoing tendencies in human organisms. Ongoing processes of recall and insight are facilitated when dissociating tendencies or "selective inattention" are held at a minimum by what is offered in the nursing situation. Sullivan defines these two aspects of the "self system" as follows:[2] *A "dissociating tendency" may be said to be at work when an event or the feelings connected with it are denied existence in awareness, even though someone else may recog-*

[2] Patrick Mullahy, *Oedipus: Myth and Complex* (New York, Hermitage House, Inc., 1948), pp. 299-300.

nize and point out what seems to be the motivation for an act. The individual cannot see what is referred to because it is not an active part of the self that operates in awareness. What is referred to has been dissociated, or pushed out of awareness, as a way of avoiding anxiety, and it is kept there for the same reason. Admitting such events or feelings into awareness would give rise to severe anxiety and thus disorganize personality. All individuals use dissociating tendencies in some degree; a pathological degree of operation of this tendency can be seen when more and more experiences and feelings are relegated to what Sullivan calls the "not-me." [3]

"Selective inattention" is referred to as a tendency in which an individual fails to notice, or to pay attention, to aspects of experience. It operates when security is threatened and requires paying strict attention to getting approval and to getting or avoiding disapproval. All else is inattended as neat discriminations are made on those aspects of experience that restore feelings of security. Selectively inattended aspects of experience continue to operate outside of "discriminated awareness." [4] However, if someone else were to mention inattended aspects of experience they can be recalled and accepted by the self. In contrast, dissociated aspects of experience are not readily subject to recall and require skillful therapeutic intervention so that the anxiety generated in the process of bringing such experiences into awareness can be held within tolerable limits.

Sullivan would conceptualize anxiety on a continuum, something in this fashion:[5]

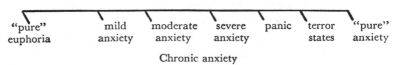

| "pure" euphoria | mild anxiety | moderate anxiety | severe anxiety | panic | terror states | "pure" anxiety |

Chronic anxiety

Fig. 8. "Polar constructs" and varying degrees of anxiety, conceptualized on a continuum, according to Sullivan.

[3] *Ibid.,* p. 294.
[4] *Ibid.,* p. 299.
[5] *Ibid.,* p. 292.

In the experience cited at the opening of this chapter it was possible to see the development of anxiety from mild to moderate degrees, and the changes in interaction between nurse and patient that took place as anxiety developed. The reader has been referred to an experience discussed earlier (p. 66) in which the account of the patient at the time of illness showed almost complete absence of anxiety, but fifteen years later selectively inattended and dissociated elements are still at work. This leads to the question: What can be done about anxiety in situations where nurses wish to be useful to patients in terms of their future development as persons? Several principles illuminate what is involved.

When anxiety is held within tolerable limits it can be a "functionally effective element in interpersonal relations." [6, 7] It is a response to unknown danger that is felt, experienced as discomfort, and that arms the human organism for mobilizing resources to meet the difficulty. Thus, it can be viewed as an aspect of the first step in solving problems, namely, the "felt need" leading to a concentration of resources. Anxiety at first alerts the individual; he can then take more facets of a situation into account. If the needed help is forthcoming and the patient can experience a strengthening of his relatedness to others because of the manner in which help is given, the personality and its resources are directed outward in a forward attack in the identification of the difficulty.

Another characteristic of anxiety as it increases in severity is the narrowing of perceptual awareness that occurs. The forces available are focused upon a smaller area of living —the difficulty that is felt. This narrowing down of what is observed permits the patient to concentrate on the problem and when skills are available for his use, to use this natural phenomenon to his own advantage.

---

[6] Sullivan, op. cit., p. 10.
[7] Edmund F. Walker, "Inducing Anxiety as Part of the Therapeutic Method," Journal of Nervous and Mental Diseases, 109:233-39 (March, 1949).

The discomfort is intensified and the area concentrated upon becomes narrowed to a crippling degree when anxiety moves toward severe anxiety or panic. The patient sees less and takes less and less into account in considering what is happening. His ability to observe what is happening and to make use of past experience in evaluating present events gives way to overfocalization on the discomfort itself. There is gross inability to consider his own feelings, the problem, the facts, the evidence, and the situation in which he finds himself. *Perceptual narrowing is minimal and alertness is increased when anxiety is of mild degree and this, in effect, accounts for its usefulness in solving problems.* In severe anxiety the view of the difficulty is greatly narrowed and alertness is reduced; any nurse who has observed the insidious development of severe anxiety has also observed, and can verify empirically, that useful learning does not, as a rule, take place.

If the nurse considers these hypotheses about anxiety she will want to know: What are the observable differences in behavior or in the subjective reports of patients or nurses when the underlying anxiety is mild and when it is of severe degree? [8, 9] What are the factors in my relationship to the patient that provoke anxiety in him, forcing him into learning that is useful or adaptation that is harmful? Since the newly admitted patient in any hospital or agency usually experiences anxiety in some degree, whether overt symptoms are manifested or not, how can I make use of that initial anxiety to facilitate positive learning for the patient during the orientation period?

Mild anxiety underlies such observable irritations as restlessness, sleeplessness, idling hostility, belittling, misunder-

[8] See for example: D. Ewen Cameron, "Some Relationships between Excitement, Depression, and Anxiety," *American Journal of Psychiatry*, Vol. 102, No. 3 (November, 1945), pp. 385-93, especially tables of symptoms.

[9] For physical concomitants see: Walter B. Cannon, *Bodily Changes in Pain, Hunger, Fear, and Rage* (New York, Appleton-Century-Crofts, Inc., 1936). H. Flanders Dunbar, *Emotions and Bodily Changes* (New York, Columbia University Press, 1935).

standings, and the like. It underlies such persisting behavior as curiosity, repetitive questioning, constant seeking of attention, reassurance, or approval. It is increased in interpersonal relationships that are perceived as threats to personal prestige, to feelings of worth, dignity, and self-respect.[10] There are infinite ways in which the nurse relating to a patient is made anxious, or, in which the patient is made to feel discomfort, each arousing in the other an older pattern of anxiety on the basis of perceptions of "real" or "illusory" events that occurred in the past but that now operate to distort interpersonal relations.

Insomnia or wakefulness in a patient may be associated with anxiety generated by a new psychological experience that is perceived as separation from a loved one, or it may be an expression of hostile feelings toward the family or nurse which have been called to mind on retiring. Thinking about such small details as inconsistencies about his dinner tray, being forced to eat, being asked or ignored on questions about bowel functions, or nurse comments on attitudes toward cleanliness may call out anxiety.[11] The additional and extra attention directed toward a wakeful patient, ensuring him of the "sustaining thereness" of the night nurse, is a way of meeting the patient's expectations and therefore of helping him to keep anxiety within tolerable limits. A nurse offering food or a snack, being symbolically interpreted in the mind of the patient as affectionate interest from a mother surrogate, is often reassuring to the patient. It demonstrates the nurse's interest in a way that words cannot convey; not infrequently sleep intervenes quickly thereafter.

In attempting to present a picture of what is involved in an experience, Sullivan accounts for anxiety as follows:[12] *Tensions, and the transformation of energy provided by*

[10] Sullivan, *op. cit.*, p. 11.

[11] See: Lowell S. Selling, "Behavior Problems of Eating," *American Journal of Orthopsychiatry*, Vol. XVI, No. 1, pp. 163-69. L. S. Selling and M. A. S. Ferraro, *The Psychology of Diet and Nutrition* (New York, W. W. Norton & Company, Inc., 1946).

[12] Sullivan, *op. cit.*, Table 1, p. 4.

tensions, constitute experience. General needs, zonal needs, and anxiety give rise to tension that is converted into overt or covert action. Various degrees of tension and anxiety have already been pointed out. It would seem from these hypotheses, and from the observations of many professional persons in the field of psychiatry, that *the purpose in offering help to an individual undergoing tension would be to aid him in making energy transformations in the direction of productive action and personality expansion.* A number of principles that guide nursing practice have already been covered and can be reviewed here to support the *hypothesis* that; *nurses face the task of developing experiences with patients that aid them to discriminate aspects of a total experience, to understand what is happening in their relations with nurses, and to develop ways that convert tension and anxiety into purposeful action.*[13] Since all symptoms are purposeful on the patient's terms, what is meant here is the ever expanding use of native endowment and capacities in the direction of self-expansion in larger social terms.

A review of guiding principles already stated in previous chapters are:

1. Instinctual drives, such as hunger, thirst, sexuality, and acquired needs, such as for belonging, for participating and contributing in order to reinforce self-respect and gain recognition from others, are imperative human needs.
2. Imperative human needs lead to tension and/or the accumulation of energy derived from tension and demand tension reduction. The reduction of tension by *any means* is felt as a reward, as satisfaction, as security or relief from discomfort, or as pleasure.
3. Tension, and the energy it provides, can be discharged in active or passive participant behavior and/or it can be partially or wholly bound within the organism as a way of avoiding felt consequences of behavior that cannot spontaneously be engaged in; it is governed by appraisals

[13] See also: Chapters 4, 8, 9, 10, 11.

of behavior made in the past by others but acting still as barriers to spontaneity.

4. When the energy of tension is bound, as in a "symptom" or a "symptomatic act," rewards and relief are felt, in the same manner that they are when tension is reduced through constructive action. (Thus consideration must be given not only to relief from tension but to the patterns and skills one uses in tackling or avoiding the difficulty that gave rise to the tension.)

5. Tension demands changes in personality and in the movement of an organism. Forward movement occurs when overt action is focused upon learning as it utilizes the energy; blocking or ineffective use of adaptive patterns of behavior occurs when channels for discharge are not visualized, as in overactivity, or are not open and/or available, as in underactivity, in the service of personality.

6. Tackling the difficulty, overriding the difficulty, and avoiding the problem altogether are patterns for converting the energy of tension into the rewards of *satisfaction* or the relief felt with safety or *security*.

7. Satisfaction is felt when an individual knows what he wants, when activities are organized for achieving clearly visualized goals that he holds in front of him. Wants imply being *for* something, seeking, struggling, striving to achieve something that is desirable.

8. Safety or security is felt when an individual orients his goals in terms of what is *not wanted*, in terms of making up for lacks, longings, deprivations that have been felt in the past, in terms of feeling less threatened, less powerless, less helpless, less anxious than he has felt in the past.

9. Often security must be felt before satisfaction can be sought.

10. Any interference to, blocking of, or barrier to an aroused need after activity toward that goal has been started and before satisfaction and/or security has been felt is perceived as frustration and reacted to by aggression, that is direct or indirect, that is, overt or covert.

11. Actions can be directed toward identifying interferences and their effects upon set goals and thus, in terms of experience, lead to variations and changes in the goal. Tension may also be reduced by giving up the goal and the satisfaction or security anticipated, or by developing fixed responses through reinforcement of dynamisms of defense that operate to defend the self without giving up the goal or the response.

12. All human behavior is purposeful and goal seeking; it is energized by tension and anxiety; it is designed wittingly or unwittingly in terms of how an individual perceives himself in relation to others and in terms of skills and abilities that he brings into play when his personality is threatened and requires that he defend himself. These behaviors require transformation of energy derived from tension and/or anxiety.

The transformation of energy derived from tension or anxiety is an ongoing human tendency; it is a way in which the human organism moves, and changes, and grows, or defends itself. The twelve principles just summarized apply to both nurse and patient. Both nurse and patient respond in relation to how they perceive themselves as well as how they perceive others in the situation.[14] When the nurse understands what is going on in a situation and when she can take this principle into account anxiety is likely to be kept at a minimum. When a nurse cannot identify her own preconceptions and expectations of patients and does not permit theirs to operate until they can communicate and develop common goals that are fully understood by each, anxiety is likely to develop and often to convert into severe degree or panic.

Personality is always organized along more or less productive lines. During *panic*, however, it disorganizes quite

[14] Donald Snygg and Arthur Combs, *Individual Behavior* (New York, Harper & Brothers, 1949). The entire text discusses, expands, and illustrates this principle of perception of self and others.

rapidly and a new reorganization follows.[15, 16] The new organization may be an improvement; it is more likely that it will be along pathological lines. A patient undergoing severe anxiety or panic cannot co-operate or collaborate with the nurse. All that can be done is to remain with the patient, to become the focus for expressed hostile remarks as a way of providing a tangible point in the patient's field toward which, however hostile, his relationship may be oriented. Listening, reflecting back to the patient what is said, responding with alacrity to requests for physical needs provide the patient with a sustaining relationship during *his* crises and provide the nurse with an opportunity to learn something about what can be done during extreme discomfort or distress. A measure of security is provided in the "thereness" of the nurse. If she can appreciate what is happening and not catch the anxiety that is being communicated to her to an extent that limits her ability to function, the panic will subside. Panic may require the presence of a professional nurse for an hour or more, doing nothing but staying with the patient and listening to what is said and responding to specific requests. Leaving the patient alone during a crisis is to reinforce the aspect of aloneness, of unrelatedness to others who must be counted upon for support, in time of need. Constant nursing participation that is cognizant of what is going on may aid the patient to reorganize personality along productive lines.

That recognition of cues to anxiety is important is illustrated in the following experience. A young woman who had previously been hospitalized for a psychotic episode had long-term psychotherapeutic assistance and later decided to become pregnant. Throughout pregnancy she felt reasonably comfortable with the idea of becoming a mother. During her hospitalization prior to delivery, however, she began to have

[15] H. S. Sullivan, *Conceptions of Modern Psychiatry* (Washington, D.C., William Alanson White Psychiatric Foundation, 1947).

[16] Flanders H. Dunbar, *Emotions and Bodily Changes* (New York, Columbia University Press, 1935). Has shown that when psychogenic death occurs it is usually related to the state of excitement that exists for the patient.

many doubts about her ability to undergo the event. Many patients were "yelling" on the ward and she wondered what that was about. No one outlined what was expected of her or the steps that she could anticipate would be followed in the delivery of her child. During delivery, nurses and doctors spoke of her *as if* she were unaware of what was happening. Their jargon frightened her and when there was disagreement about the position of the infant's head, she became more and more uncomfortable. Finally the delivery was over and she was returned to her room. When she asked whether she could see her baby (in order to find out if its head was all right) she was told that she would have to wait for twenty-four hours. Her anxiety mounted with each relationship with professional personnel. Finally, she realized partly what was going on and decided that she ought to talk it over with one of the nurses. She decided to ask the nurse for a bedpan and if the nurse looked interested in her she would discuss her discomfort. The nurse said, "You will have to wait until we pass them one hour from now." Her anxiety moved swiftly and the next day she was removed to a psychiatric hospital for a second psychotic episode.

Anxiety can be communicated by visitors, as is shown in the following experience: Mrs. Brown lived with her husband's family and described her mother-in-law to the nurse as a person who could not make a mistake. Throughout her pregnancy her mother-in-law found fault with what Mrs. Brown did; she didn't dress properly, she didn't eat properly, she couldn't take care of herself, etc. Later, Mrs. Brown entered a maternity hospital, had an uneventful delivery, and seemed very happy about the outcome until it was time to talk about going home. On being informed that the date had been set she expressed fear and inability in taking care of her baby. How would she handle it, feed it, bathe it; these were things she could not do. All of the former appraisals made by her mother-in-law seemed to go into operation at once. The nurse was busy but she could see that Mrs. Brown was greatly concerned. She quickly rearranged her schedule and sat down to listen. The patient cried and the nurse said, "You want to have a good cry, go ahead." She listened. Soon the patient came to recognize that she was saying the same things about herself that her mother-in-law had said about her. Once in awareness she could decide what the possibilities or courses of action were that she could take in her own behalf.

Developing awareness of the influence of powerful individuals who made appraisals of the patient during his past life is one way of diminishing anxiety. In developing such awareness—by permitting patients to talk out their feelings and concerns about the present illness—a nurse aids the patient to harness the energy derived from tension or anxiety to learning about living. The development of awareness of present and future goals, with relation to limitations enforced by illness, is an activity that uses energy. Planning activities and steps that are necessary for reaching goals are experiences that convert energy into productive functioning. Learning techniques and skills required for planned activities is a way of putting to use the tension or anxiety that is generated in a nursing situation. *Nurses can aid patients to convert mild anxiety into productive activity and they can observe for the development of more severe degrees of anxiety and examine their relations with patients for cues that identify the basis that is intensifying anxiety.*

It is doubtful that anxiety can be "alleviated" without knowing what is going on in the nurse and patient relationship; it is questionable whether attempts at *quick relief* for anxiety are more useful than attempting to *harness the energy* into activity that develops skills useful in future relations with people. If a nurse has developed ability to undergo tension and stress, in order to identify a difficulty that she feels and to take steps that lead to a course of action based on evidence of what is involved, she will be able to help patients to do likewise. A nurse learns these skills by working through her own problems and concerns that arise in her relations with others. Aiding nurses to learn the process of tackling human problems, including their own, is a task of every basic professional school. May[17] emphasizes that the capacity for creativity and the proclivity for anxiety are two sides of the same capacity and that both interlock and operate together in the development of awareness of discrepancies between what is expected and what is experienced in reality. The power to overcome difficulties of many sorts lies in bringing expectations and reality together through a process of transforming both, and as a result of using the energy provided by tension.

Anxiety and guilt

Guilt is a feeling that is perceived when the way an individual views himself is inadequate to the new situation. If there is a discrepancy between the concept of self [18] and the actions or performances in a given situation, the individual is likely to feel guilty. He may or may not express it in words. Guilt is related to lacks perceived as being in the self, errors in judgment that are made, and actions that are recognized as inappropriate to a situation. Guilt often leads to attempts at reparation, such as self-punishment, self-recrimination, expiation, and the like.

Guilt is related to tendencies that operate outside awareness, tendencies that have not been evaluated and fully understood, that could not be brought into the focus of attention when parental disapproval was felt and when approval in a situation was earnestly sought. Guilt calls out anxiety as a reminder to the individual that personality and its needs are threatened. It may also call out the expectation of punishment that, during childhood, was meted out by parents who took on this responsibility for the child's management. In

---

[17] Rollo May, *The Meaning of Anxiety* (New York, The Ronald Press, 1950), p. 356. In the writer's opinion this is the best single reference source on principles of anxiety—its nature and its consequences.
[18] See Chapter 10.

adulthood, when parental punishment is no longer forthcoming, self-punishment operates through the incorporated parental injunctions against shortcomings and failures. Thus, new situations continue to be evaluated and controlled by parental "images" which communicate threats that lead to perception of guilt and anxiety.

Since recognition of failure to meet approved standards conflicts with the need for self-enhancement, secrecy is most often connected with feelings of guilt.[19] Security is gained through secrecy, rather than through revealing to others what is felt. Perhaps one of the most noticeable occurrences of guilt and secrecy occurs in students; lacks in knowledge are rarely revealed and when it is required—as in presenting a paper to an instructor or a class—severe anxiety may be felt. Yet, when the discrepancy is finally revealed and the student and instructor are both aware of gaps in knowledge required to understand problems, the way is opened for growth and progress. Guilt and its intensification give rise to anxiety that can be used to further learning or that can be intensified so that defenses against threat are used in order to feel secure. But, guilt itself is a luxury that restricts an individual and limits the attention that can be given to what is going on in a situation.

Most often, guilt operates outside awareness; it may be observed in actions rather than in what is said. Minute cues to the need for self-punishment offer leads for protecting the patient against this need. Such cues may be in the nature of asking to be hurt, asking that services be denied, refusing to work toward comfort. They may be in the nature of other data, such as poems about death, pictures about gruesome events, or great interest in lurid tales of suicide in the newspapers. In depressions and suicidal attempts these cues may be seen full blown, engaging many actions of the individual. Partial resolution of guilt is inferred in psychosomatic evi-

---

[19] Snygg, *op. cit.*, elaborates what is involved in the need for self-enhancement as it operates for all individuals.

dence, such as vomiting, pleading for bitter medications or repeated enemas, when these are not required by the medical problem. These are all ways of expiating guilt.

Self-punishment helps the individual to save face and it often brings the needed attention despite failure; thus, it may also function as a stepping stone to growth—what is offered can be accepted as earlier debts are paid. Growth requires recognition of feelings that produce guilt and identification of their relation to what is expected in a situation. It requires exploration of feelings that lead to a new view of self. Perhaps the best discussion of self-harm or self-punishment is given by Menninger[20] who points out the strength of "the wish to die." Many patients who otherwise have a seemingly good chance for medical recovery seem to validate Menninger's hypotheses; their behavior seems to be organized and to operate in a way that suggests negation of life and living. Symonds has also reviewed the literature on this subject and provided a comprehensive discussion of guilt.[21]

Masochism is a form of self-punishment in which more or less complete physical or psychological destruction of self seems to be preferred as a defense against further threats to the self and as a way of shifting responsibility for growth and change to others.[22] Punishment is sought, the self is felt to be unworthy, suffering and pity are courted as ways of enhancing the self. Recognition of suffering in others and sublimating all of one's own needs into activities designed to relieve that suffering, in martyrlike fashion, are ways of overcoming and assuaging one's own guilt feelings.

From the standpoint of nursing patients, recognition of the force inherent in guilt is necessary. All protective aspects of

[20] K. A. Menninger, *Man against Himself* (New York, Harcourt Brace & Company, 1938) and *Love against Hate* (New York, Harcourt Brace & Company, 1942).

[21] Percival Symonds, *Dynamics of Human Adjustment* (New York, Appleton-Century-Crofts, Inc., 1946).

[22] Theodore Reik, *Masochism in Modern Man* (New York, Farrar & Rinehart, Inc., 1941); Erich Fromm, *Escape from Freedom* (New York, Farrar & Rinehart, Inc., 1941) and "Selfishness and Self-love," *Psychiatry*, 2:507-523 (1938).

care require recognition of tendencies toward self-punishment and early alertness to minute cues that indicate contemplated self-destruction. Often such cues require highly developed discriminative judgment and close attention to ordinary behavior that seems all right. A patient is reading a poem about death and although previously depressed he now appears more relaxed; the next day his suicidal jump is announced in the papers. A patient draws a picture of two inert figures lying on the ground and the next day attempts to harm herself. It is probable that there are almost always cues to future behavior that nurses can observe and that attention concentrated on identifying them is of greater value than wholesale watching of all depressed patients.

A nurse cannot pay attention to cues in the situation when her own needs are uppermost and require attention in the situation. Her observations are, unwittingly, focused upon the way in which her unrecognized needs are being met by a patient. A good deal of advice has been given to nurses on how to behave in relation to patients; it is a rare book that points out, in addition, the fact that the nurse may generate anxiety and guilt when her own needs operate outside awareness and are not met by patients. However, *until the actual needs of the nurse are met or identified so that she is aware of what they are and how they function as barriers to the patient's goals,* she does not have control such as is required for carrying out all of the "shoulds" and "musts" indicated in nursing literature. She cannot gain rapport with patients when her own anxiety restricts awareness and limits her attention and observation to what brings approval for her. A few examples will suffice to show the manner in which unrecognized needs acted as barriers to the study and improvement of interpersonal relations in nursing, in particular instances where nurses were investigating their relations with patients in order to find out what was actually going on:

1. "It was apparent from his facial expression that he resented being brought in for such purpose (talking to the

nurse) and did not quite believe my explanation for it."
(Later) "If you want me to, I will have the supervisor
assign me to someone else and you can go out."

Note the anticipatory tension and the nurse's anxiety that
led to a need to avoid the contact, but expressed as pseudo-
consideration of the patient's wishes.

2. "Things seemed to be going my way so I could afford to
   relax."

This is a direct expression of the fact that the nurse in this
situation is not anxious because her expectations are being
met.

3. (At the beginning) "I unconsciously tried to impress the
   patient and attempted to differentiate myself from hospital
   personnel." (Later) "Time was short and I wanted to do
   well and quickly." (Later, the patient) "You are a nice
   nurse." (Directly after, the nurse) "I am surprised to find
   that I like her and wish I could in some way help her."

The nurse in this report manages her anxiety by attempting
to ensure her individuality, thus expressing a need for prestige. Time factors and the need for quick success interfere
with rapport and may lead to feelings of guilt. When the
nurse's needs were met and the patient indicated interest
the anxiety abated and the relationship proceeded along
helpful lines.

These excerpts from reports, and others indicated in this
text, are examples of honest reporting of the performances in
interpersonal events. While they point out that nurses have
ego needs and that failure to meet them leads to anxiety and
to feelings of guilt, they also have shown that when nurses
become more fully aware of their needs they no longer operate to interfere with what is going on in their relations with
patients. An individual does not feel secure in revealing to
others tendencies in himself about which he feels guilty.
"Shoulds" and "musts" in nursing education make it more
difficult for nurses to reveal to themselves and to others what

they actually feel in a situation. Yet, *identifying what is actually felt is a sound guarantee of the development of persons in nursing who will want to nurse patients and who will be able to take on the task of self-nurture in the future.* It provides a basis for developing nursing practices that can be carried out willingly, intelligently, and with satisfaction by a nurse who knows what she observes, understands its meanings, and can base her actions upon observation and understanding.

Anxiety and doubt

Doubts frequently arise in the minds of patients. They ask: "Am I going to come out of this all right?" "I'm not sure my doctor can do this job." "That nurse isn't doing it right." Doubts arise when activity incurs indecision, as in conflict, or when barriers to goals are perceived, as in frustration. The anxiety generated is always in relation to interpersonal relations with either nurses or individuals for whom nurses stand. It may be mild to severe in degree. Severe anxiety occurs when a patient does not have in his repertoire of behavior a method permitting himself to doubt what is occurring, or when there is "wholesale" doubting of everything, or when his doubts do not lead to clarification of what is involved in the problem under consideration.

What a patient believes to be true about his medical problem may lead to a state so comfortable and so secure that he may not be able successfully to withstand new developments. This phenomenon can be observed, particularly, if his convictions operate on the basis of need for quick relief from anxiety and doubt, rather than full consideration of evidence available to him.

The question of doubting ideas is important for nurses, too. For example, those nurses who received their basic nursing education many years ago learned, in Pediatrics, that each child must be put on a rigid schedule of feeding, sleeping, and toilet training. The extreme position is well illustrated in the reference cited below.[23] In contrast, those nurses who served during World War II, in the Army Nurse Corps, and were in the vicinity where an entirely different child-rearing pattern was in operation, as reported by Moloney,[24] were in a position to examine new evidence on relationships of mother and child. Infants in Okinawa were exposed to considerable permissiveness in relation to feeding, toilet training, and the like.

Unless a nurse has some doubts about the validity of present practices in education, and the subject matter of nursing inquiry, she will be unable to consider both reports cited above in the light of all available evidence including recent reports with regard to "self-demand feeding," "rooming-in," and the like. That is, she will have a system of attitudes and beliefs on infant care and, being unable to permit or to undergo doubt in relation to ideas held, will continue to operate uncritically under ideas learned many years ago. *Ideas and principles are guides to action and it is only as they are held open to review and reconstruction that new practices in nursing can be evolved.* The future of nursing is not fixed; rational doubt is to be viewed as legitimate rebellion against the *status quo* leading progressively and creatively to the reconstruction of patterns of activity.

The question always arises as to whether nurses should *allay doubt* expressed by patients or whether they should assist the patient to *undergo doubt,* as a necessary condition for identifying, formulating, and tackling the problems at hand. The issue is largely dependent upon the nurse's ability to recognize anxiety and to assist patients in its management through intelligent methods of inquiry. As resource persons nurses aid patients to become acquainted with facts, and with sources to facts, connected with medical ailments peripheral to the central problem. However, nurses often face problems related to assisting patients to examine feelings of doubt

---

[23] U.S. Govt. Publication No. 8, Children's Bureau, 1940, p. 3.

[24] James Clark Moloney, "Psychiatric Observations in Okinawa Shima," *Psychiatry,* 8:391-99 (November, 1945).

regarding the feelings a patient has for others—his family, friends, fellow workers, other nurses, doctors, as well as others cultural figures. *Nurses can recognize the anxiety factor inherent in doubt and permit expression of feelings, aiding the patient to see what the situation means to him, without interrogating for information.* If questions are asked they can be open-ended so as to lead the patient to re-examine what he has felt and to allow him to arrive at his own conclusions on courses of action.

For example, a doctor and two staff nurses have repeatedly informed a patient that he is going to recover from his present illness. Each time that he indicates his own feelings about his present predicament by saying, "I won't pull through this," these workers assure him that he will get well. After several days, during which the patient's feelings about his present situation have not changed despite reassurance, he commented to another nurse that he didn't think that his doctor or the two nurses in question knew what they were doing. He doubted their ability. The staff nurse merely commented, "You feel that they are in the dark about your problem." To this comment the patient responded, saying, "Yes, I have been trying to tell them that I feel the whole thing is hopeless but they will not listen to me." Now the nurse could aid this patient to focus on the core of his doubt about the ability of the doctors and nurses, namely, the interference to his expression of deeply felt convictions about himself and his present dilemma. The nurse did not point out to the patient the omnipotence of the physician or the other two nurses but rather focused upon aiding the patient to learn something about himself that would make it possible for him to clarify his need to doubt professional abilities in others.

When nurses are placed in the position of assisting patients to undergo doubts connected with social and ethical concepts, they gain considerable assistance from members of the professional team in developing methods for helping patients therapeutically in these respects. While nurses exemplify in their behavior the highest social and ethical insights and values of a culture, their concern is not with imposing these values on others. The nursing process involves use of methods and provision of conditions that make it possible for any patient to re-evaluate and reconstruct his own beliefs and attitudes, and to discover new ones through social institutions or resources of his own choosing other than nursing. The nursing process is open-ended; it does not impose values and standards; it aids others to examine the evidence and to arrive at discriminated judgments on their own decisions. The need for interprofessional assistance is implied in the following study of a relationship between nurse and patient.

Nurse	*Patient*	*Comment*
"Hello, I'm Miss ———."	"Hello."	
"What are you doing in bed?"	"Oh, I didn't feel well yesterday. My stomach was upset and I couldn't eat."	The patient probably empathized that the nurse preferred that he got out of bed.
"Do you feel better now?"	"Yes but I can't get up yet."	
"Do you mind if I sit down?"	"Not at all."	
"Do you feel like talking?"	"Yes, by talking I might help others to get better."	Note that he thinks talking will help others; infers that it may not help him.
"Why did you come here?"	"About six months ago I went to the ——— (cleric) to talk to him. He wasn't home and the lady there kicked me out."	The religious identity of the cleric is omitted in this report.
"Why did she do that?"	"I couldn't figure it out, I hadn't been fresh or anything."	
"Why do you think she kicked you out?"	"I don't know."	Note the number of times the patient says, "I don't know." The nurse bombards him with questions but offers no assistance in clarifying.
"What happened then?"	"I hung around for a while and then I went	

Nurse	Patient	Comment
	home. I couldn't sleep and around 4.00 A.M. I telephoned the (cleric).	
(With the patient's answer I came to feel that he was quite suspicious.)	He answered immediately. He said I got him out of bed, but if he was in bed, how come he answered the phone so quick, and he didn't sound like he was sleeping."	This perception of "felt relations" by the nurse was verified by the patient's readiness to read into the facts, rather than to delay his judgments until more facts were known.
"What did he say?" "What happened next?"	(No answer.) "I went back to see him and he kicked me out."	Note that the nurse is using direct questions and is not working for continuity and clarity of ideas expressed, but is getting information which she does not use in a helpful way.
"Why would a (cleric) do that?"	"That's what I wondered. Guess it was because I hadn't been to church."	
"Clerics don't usually kick people out."	"I believe religion is like science, there has to be a supreme power. I got all mixed up thinking about Jews, Catholics, and Protestants."	
"How do you feel about it now?" (I wondered why this patient was showing so much doubt. I almost felt that I wanted to tell him he was wrong.)	"I don't know. I don't know if there is a God."	This is a cue to the fact that this patient is unclear in apprehending the meaning of the concept of God.
"Yes" (gave the patient a cigarette).	"Do you have a cigarette?"	
"What happened when the cleric kicked you out?"	"I went home and called the cops, and started to cry. They took me to the hospital."	Note the impotant rage and the calling on another authority when one failed to give help that was needed. Two questions in one attacks the patient's defenses, note the growing unclearness of his remarks.
"Why did you cry and why did they take you to the hospital?"	"I don't know if they were cops."	

Nurse	*Patient*
"Why do you say that?"	"I never looked at the cops uniform closely enough to tell. I don't know if he was a cleric, either."
"Why would they be dressed as cops and clerics if they weren't?"	"I don't know."

The purpose in presenting this material is to show that the question of doubt comes up in nursing; it is not meant to advocate interrogation as method useful to the patient. It does show that nurses face the recurring problem of patient's questioning their faith in others and their social and ethical beliefs and that *a method that permits the patient to explore his doubts and feelings and to discover what his convictions are is indicated.* It also shows the need for interprofessional relations with allied professional workers, such as members of various clergy.

Anxiety and phobias, obsessions, and compulsions

In the face of fear and anxiety, which involve real and/or unknown dangers to personality, many "coping mechanisms" are used. Among them are phobias, obsessions, and compulsions which are responses that assure avoidance of an object or situation thought to represent the danger. The anticipatory nature of these avoidance responses is an outstanding feature. The danger of an object or an event originally experienced as connected with a concrete experience now becomes an expectation or anticipation of danger that is transferred to objects or events that have not yet been experienced by the individual. Thus, tendencies to avoid new experiences limit the individual's participation and inhibit his movement in the direction of finding out about and judging each new experience on its own merits. An ill-defined, remote experience in which fear and anxiety were felt in severe degree, often functions as a criterion for judging all future experience. Consequently, the task in nursing patients who respond in terms of nonrational fears, such as phobias, obsessions, and/or compulsions, is to assist the patient to learn to undergo each new experience in the nursing situation in the simplest, most easily understandable terms. There is need also to develop methods for evaluating the event in progress, on its own terms, as it is being undergone.

A *phobia* represents an acquired need to avoid stressful situations. The inability of the patient to connect his present phobic response with the stress that actually caused it serves to protect against anxiety connected with an awareness of difficulties not met in an earlier situation. Since the perception that produces anxiety is a view of self as inadequate or helpless in the face of need to cope with crises, there is need to exclude it from awareness.[25] Two purposes are thus served: the self is assured that help will be forthcoming from others and the self is protected against further recognition of its inadequacies. Self-enhancement is served; this is particularly true when phobias are associated with an illness that is socially accepted as a way of expressing helplessness and getting desired assistance.

The purposive aspect of phobias operates outside awareness and the patient is not conscious of the process nor is he able to exercise control over his responses until he has examined, with a competent psychotherapist, the underlying feelings of self and of relatedness to others. These feelings concerning others—often expectations of injury from them and feelings of hostility and domination over them—are directly related to the view of self that is held. Perceiving himself as helpless requires that all assistance in meeting daily events and crises must largely come from outside the self, from others. Acting out dependency longings upon others is assured since the self cannot act in its own behalf. Fear and

[25] See Chapter 10.

anxiety are displaced upon objects and persons other than the self. By avoiding them the experience of fear or anxiety is avoided.

Phobias develop in children, when their self-esteem is devastatingly threatened. Unless the child has other opportunities for expanding his concept of self, and of others, and of the world, in a comfortable and secure way, phobias may develop in more and more areas of life and consolidate into one rigid phobia.

For example, a three-year-old child intimidated by a six-year-old is told that she should be careful in taking a bath for she will slip down the drain. The three-year-old, for reasons to be found in her current mother-father-child relationship, is most unclear about her perception of self and has many feelings of inadequacy. Consequently, she soon expresses disinterest in taking a bath, without expressing that she has been made to feel afraid of losing a part of herself down the drain. The observer recognized the possibility that the dynamics at work might lead to the development of a more rigid phobia. In terms of assisting the child to examine her own experience with the drain, and to find out whether it was possible to slip down the drain, the observer began with some soap and later paints which were used as play materials in the sink. When appropriate moments of "good feeling" were noted in the observer-child relationship, the child was helped to express and to clarify her feelings about slipping down the drain. This required a long period of time and a sustaining relationship that was gradually strengthened. Finally, the child was able to climb into the tub (which was never demanded while she was afraid of it) and to "find out for myself" whether it was possible to slip down the drain. In finding out that this was quite impossible, a new perception of self took place, as indicated in the child's assertion, "I don't have to be afraid of that old drain. I tried it and I can't go down if I wanted to." When the observer remarked, "You mean you checked up to find out whether the drain could hurt you?" the child replied, "Yes, and I know it can't, and I found out for myself that Mary was wrong."

The important element in the example above is that the child has not substituted the observer's knowledge for her own. She has in this instance learned and made use of a method of inquiry as further safeguard against the development of other irrational fears pending the strengthening of her own self-concept. This kind of learning is made possible when her need for security is permitted to operate and at the same time a nonjudgmental relationship is offered, which lead her to doubt her own actions and to arrive at some conclusions about them.

It is necessary to keep in mind that patients in a situation often take in both content and method from nurses, but that *the most important learning*—that which leads to understandings which will influence forward movement—*has to do with developing skills to use methods.* When adulthood has been reached, without the development of such methods as examining each situation or event on its own merits, the strength of a phobia is likely to be such that intensive psychotherapy will not always be successful. Psychotherapy of all kinds requires that the patient be able to undergo the anxiety connected with self-examination, as well as to inquire into the actual facts of the present situation with the sustaining assistance of the therapist. An outstanding feature seen in patients who, seeking safety, use phobias to integrate interpersonal situations is their inability to express doubt.

For example, a man aged sixty-seven has been largely a dependent individual all of his life. His wife tended him carefully, demanding very little for herself, waiting on his every need—feeding him promptly, buying his clothes, laying out what he should wear to work, and the like. Shortly after the death of his wife, the man was retired, receiving a small pension from his employers. This pension largely represented security in that he would now be able to live without being a financial burden to others—a situation to be avoided.

However, soon it became apparent that his needs for unconditional dependence were not being met by people, that it was necessary for him to buy food, to prepare it, to decide what to wear, and the like. Gradually, vague symptoms developed—such as falling on the street and in other ways requiring help from others in a way that seemed more legitimate than asking directly for it. He became fearful and began to walk less and less, assuring others that he could not take care of himself because of these physical concomitants of old age. These falls were never evaluated in a medical way—a physician was never consulted to find out whether they were of physical origin or what could be done to prevent them. They were made use of as a way of rationalizing feelings of helplessness that stemmed from his perception of himself and as a way of assuring that others in the situation would watch over him in an unconditional way. The longings for dependency may have been connected with expectations of abandonment, an expectation that arises in childhood and in this instance has probably not been worked through. When others take responsibility for meeting problems connected with existence for the remaining days of life he is assured that his expectations of abandonment are false and that his longings will be met. One can speculate on the wisdom of lifelong, unconditional care that has trapped him and reinforced his feelings of helplessness; it is likely that giving it filled a need held by his wife—a need of which she, too, was unaware.

Psychotherapy for this aged man holds little hope for bringing safely into awareness the underlying perception of self and recognition of the longing for unconditional care. Anxiety has long been pinned down in his way of life. From the standpoint of nursing, definitive care would include meeting his longing for help and observing for cues that show a wish for self-expansion. There is the possibility that further growth is limited in most individuals who have reached this point in life with so meager a view of self-initiated action.

Anxiety and obsessions and compulsions

Obsessions are usually thought of as ideas that dominate and limit the possibility of new experiences bringing about a revision in thinking. They express acquired needs or longings, or there may be feelings that constrict experience. There is always limited recognition in awareness of the origin of these barriers to further growth and hence expression is usually indirect. Thus, actions—called "compulsive acts"—that provide a way of managing dominant thoughts that are neither acceptable nor avoidable are most often what can be observed. Obsessions and compulsions are usually seen together—the obsession being an idea or feeling that must be avoided at all costs in order to feel safe. A compulsive act is the ameliorative activity performed to manage the anxiety that would arise if the forbidden thoughts or feelings gained entrance into awareness.

Persistent thoughts that preoccupy and thus exclude other possible ideas from the mind of an individual set up internal conflict. Images, illusory of individuals important in the child's life, operate in adulthood without critical intervention of the adult; he permits these images to disapprove thoughts and feelings that arise. However, the obsessive thought cannot be entirely avoided because it also represents a wish or longing that has been dissociated; it is, in effect, his wish, his thought, his feeling, and as such, an aspect of self-expression. As in all conflict, hesitation, vacillation, and/or blocking of the actual expression of the wish may be observed. Vacillation may continue so that a decision cannot be reached; however, most individuals resolve the conflict by counteracting the obsessive thought with a compulsive act.

Obsessive thoughts and compulsive acts are a matter of degree; all individuals make use of these coping mechanisms at some time during life and in some degree. Extreme degrees may be seen in the psychiatric problems of patients who are institutionalized in psychiatric hospitals. Less extreme degrees may be seen in everyday situations in all hospitals or clinics.

If a patient is obsessed with a thought concerning germs, filth, or masturbation, connected with the use of his hands, compulsive hand-washing may keep in abeyance the obsessive wish to get his hands dirty or to masturbate with them. This sequence may be observed in nursery schools where children, ages three to six, have an already well-stereotyped idea or attitude about keeping their hands clean. These children cannot participate in finger-painting, playing with clay, and making tunnels with wet sand. If they venture expression of a wish to engage in these experiences, as some of the other children do, a look of great concern may usually be observed on their faces as they rush to the bathroom to wash their hands. The hand-washing is a security operation through which the child feels safe in the face of disapproval that has been experienced in actual relations with parents, and which is now felt in the present situation from which parents are absent. Parents have communicated rigid attitudes toward cleanliness and rewarded these children for accepting them. However, if the teacher permits the child this security, makes no comment about the inability to participate and the need to wash hands, and provides the child with real interest which expresses acceptance of him as a person, the child may begin to doubt what is happening. He may begin to structure his experiences in terms of home, where hands must be kept clean, and school, where one's wishes may be expressed freely. He may learn that different adults have different expectations of him and begin to discriminate between them.

It is important to keep in mind that the compulsive act is an adaptation that was required and reinforced in early childhood when the child was dependent upon an approving mother for satisfaction and security. When satisfactions are not permitted, life is patterned to include acts that seem to ensure security or feeling safe. Avoiding getting hands dirty is an adaptation that may spread to other areas; disapproval of wishes becomes symbolized or generalized and operates in areas such as bowel function, sexual and other creative activities, and the like. Character traits that emerge, when childhood training in these respects is excessively rigid, and where attitudes to which a child has been exposed require reinforcement of these adaptations, are: extreme orderliness, cleanliness, stubbornness, hoarding, extreme idealism often leading to excessive consideration of the wishes of others to the exclusion of self. These character traits do not always appear in pure forms but may occur in combination with opposite traits; in one aspect of life there may be extreme orderliness and in another extreme disorderliness.

Orderliness and cleanliness are desirable traits in everyone; these traits may operate in a compulsive way, as when disorder in a dayroom cannot be tolerated although that disorder is temporary and stems from activities that patients have underway. On the other hand contradictory trends may operate. A nurse may insist upon cleanliness and demand "perfect" order in her nursing sphere of activity and yet maintain her room and her educational activities in a haphazard, disorderly way. In the area of relatedness to others, a nurse may expect, indeed demand, that the patient come to understand everything on the basis of reasoning, or acceptance and compliance with precepts or ideals that are held before him, giving little recognition to the more "disorderly" manner in which feelings arise and are expressed in nonrational ways.

Obsessional ideas and compulsive acts are fixed responses, or more or less systematized ways of behaving. They represent routine or stereotyped ways of thinking and acting that are adaptations in response to threats to personality that were felt when barriers to personal wishes were perceived in earlier experiences. The inacceptable tendencies or wishes, to which barriers were raised in earlier situations, are now inacceptable but not wholly so. The basis of their inacceptability is most generally that of hostility or aggressive attack toward others, and these "real" or honest expressions of the self responding to barriers required distortion in earlier situations. In order to maintain that distortion and the illusion of safety, compulsive acts and systematized ways of thinking and acting have been reinforced in the process of growing up. In this way, it can be seen, hatred can be masked by excessive love and may operate in more or less tenuous fashion. Strivings to "do good" to "help others" replace and manage ambivalent feelings and hostility that are kept outside awareness. While this is desirable, inasmuch as hatred may operate—when unleashed—in murderous ways, it is undesirable in that the basic way of acting reinforces a denial of self. Everyone becomes angry, feels hostility, responds with aggression to barriers that block progress. Examination of these feelings in the open and the necessity for denying that they ever operate are two possibilities that can be pursued in various situations.

Thoughts and actions based upon positive affirmation of self, including recognition and conscious appraisal and redirection of the ability to feel hatred toward loved ones, is a mature accomplishment in the growing up process. It can become a possibility in a situation; it cannot be coerced as an outcome without paying the price of further distortion of experience. An important ingredient in maturity is the ability to recognize parents, teachers, and other status persons, as *individuals* rather than authorities to whom one submits. They are seen as individuals having strengths for which they are respected, and weaknesses which are understood, tolerated, and accepted as an aspect of the *person as he is.* This achievement cannot occur when hatred cannot be expressed, remains unrecognized, and is managed in so tenuous a fashion as a compulsive need to "be good." It is only when an individual can come to recognize most of the tendencies in himself—love, hatred, dependence, pride—and grow in the direction of mature expression of self as one who chooses to love, wants to relate himself to others, feels anger when the situation calls for it, and yet wishes to be productive as a person.

This choice is not open to individuals whose character is

structured to include severe obsessions and compulsions without sustained therapeutic assistance. Therapy permits the patient to undergo steps in self-examination at his own rate of speed, and in ways that lead to recognition of the pluralistic nature of human tendencies. Understanding and conscious subordination of destructive impulses that may operate against the self and others leads in the direction of affirmation of self and activities that are productive in future experiences.

Nurses cannot undertake this kind of therapy with patients. They can study the way in which coping mechanisms, such as phobias, obsessions, and compulsions, operate. Nurses can develop ways to assist patients to feel safe with them. Nurses can accept patients as they are without becoming involved in their pathology. More importantly, the recognition of the fact that obsessions, compulsions, and phobias are ways of binding anxiety leads to understanding that whatever is done must include recognition that anxiety increases gradually and insidiously when defenses are attacked. Permitting the patient's own rigid regulations that he has set for himself to operate, and to make it possible for them to operate, is a way of deepening his feelings of security possibly to a point where he will feel safe enough to doubt what he is doing. Because the anxiety is great any doubt of the validity of the patient's acts may increase his anxiety. When doubt comes from the patient it is his feeling and he will initiate actions in accordance with it; when doubt is initiated by the nurse it may function as another barrier, requiring redoubling of his efforts toward security.

For example, often at bedtime, patients will find it difficult to settle down to sleep. The patient must have the pillow beaten in a certain way, a certain number of times. The water glass and the light must be arranged in particular ways, the bed sheets must be absolutely straight—the patient feels a wrinkle although the nurse has exerted great effort to do what has been asked. These forms of behavior when studied shed light on the obsessional thoughts that they may be counteracting. Forbidden thoughts may arise as the patient is preparing to go to sleep. The patient is helpless because of illness and he expects the nurse to carry out his compulsive acts that ensure sleep. These ways of relating to the nurse may be studied in relation to the particular medical or surgical problem that brought the patient to the hospital for further treatment. They may be studied from the standpoint of the degree of diffuseness, by which they enter into the new hospital experience and the relationship with various nurses.[26, 27] Recording carefully the requests and the ways of responding to these demands of patients and their effects on the outcome of illness as an experience in learning for the patient leads to the development of sound ways of nursing patients whose character is expressed in obsessive, compulsive, or phobic manner.

Summary

Unexplained discomfort can often be recognized as anxiety, frequently coupled with guilt, doubt, fears, and obsessions. When it arises as a psychological experience connected with how the patient feels about himself in his present predicament, the nursing offered should be based upon psychological principles. Principles derived from biological and physical sciences may be interrelated with ones from psychological and social sciences in order to arrive at practices that are useful to the patient. Psychological principles have been outlined in this chapter.

Anxiety is a potent force in interpersonal relations and the energy it provides is converted into destructive or constructive action depending upon the perception and understanding of all parties in the situation. With new patients, nurses

[26] See particularly: Edward Glover, "Sublimation, Substitution, and Social Anxiety," *International Journal of Psychoanalysis* (1931), pp. 263-97.

[27] Edmund Bergler, "Psychopathology of Compulsive Smoking," *Psychiatric Quarterly*, 20:297-321 (April, 1946). Points out that the compulsive nature of smoking is often uncovered when medical limitations are placed on smoking.

can attempt to meet requests for information and assistance promptly. In so doing, they can work for clarity in understanding what each expects of the other and what preconceptions about what a nurse or a patient will do are operating. When a mutual relationship has been reached common goals that aid in the solution of the problem can be developed. Harnessing energy derived from tension and anxiety into finding out what is felt and thought about being sick or injured, and exploring goals and making plans together, helps the patient to strengthen his relations with others and thus to keep his anxiety at a minimum. Communication with patients and control of their behavior by them is more likely when the nurse is able to perceive changes in her behavior, in her expectations, in her preconceptions of what is required.[28] Reduction of anxiety and bringing about constructive changes in the patient often require examination of how the nurse feels about the patient and how the patient feels about the nurse's gestures, behavior, and words. Keeping anxiety within tolerable limits and making use of the energy it provides are nursing functions that require understanding of what is happening in the relationship, principles that illuminate the action, in order to design experiences in relationships with patients through which they can strengthen personality. Because anxiety limits the area of observation and restricts what can be focused upon to that which is in line with expectations and preconceptions, there is great need for nurse and patient to work together to find out what each is seeking in the current relationship.

[28] Snygg, *op. cit.*, p. 17.

Part III. PSYCHOLOGICAL TASKS

Purpose: *The purpose of Part III is to identify those psychological tasks encountered in the process of learning to live with people as an aspect of formation and development of personality and as an aspect of the tasks demanded of nurses in their relations with patients. These tasks will be related to ones ordinarily undergone during various developmental eras. Since illness is an event that is experienced along with feelings that derive from older experiences but are re-enacted in the relationship of nurse to patient, the nurse-patient relationship is seen as an opportunity for nurses to help patients to complete the unfinished psychological tasks of childhood in some degree. The relationship of principles discussed in Part II and of the roles discussed in Part I will be expanded and applied in discussion of psychological tasks and possible courses of action that grow out of a nurse's understanding of various situations. This section of the book will bring together all that has been discussed so far, focusing on ways that nursing can function as a maturing force in society. Development of still other ways will come from practicing nurses who find the theory outlined to be useful and from those who make subsequent revisions or changes in the theory in the light of further evidence to explain more of what goes on in nurse-patient relations.*

CHAPTER **8**

Learning to Count on Others

Overview

WHEN AN INDIVIDUAL is sick he is dependent upon others for information and care that will aid in the solution of his medical problem. The way in which he responds to the necessity of asking for and of receiving help from others depends in large measure on how he feels about himself in a situation in which he is dependent. Feelings of dependence develop very early in life, during the mother and child relationship, and are often carried forward into adulthood with little change as a result of many intervening experiences. Some individuals are able to modify adaptations and expand what is learned early in life. Nurses come into contact with people who have revised their feelings about getting help from others and those who have not. Being able to see relationships between early childhood experiences and adult behavior and between the infant's complete helplessness and that seen in comatose patients aids a nurse to make discriminations in offering care and in developing with patients experiences that will afford further personality development. The purpose of this chapter is to clarify these relationships and to identify what is involved when patients and nurses are faced with the task of learning to count on others for help.

Essential questions

What is an infant capable of feeling and deciding for himself? How does he communicate his needs to others? What are the goals of his communication? What can others do about it? To phrase these academic questions as "real" difficulties that a mother faces in her relations with an infant: What does this infant want when he cries? What kind of help does he want from me? These same problems arise in situations where nurses are offering service to comatose or otherwise completely helpless patients. It is easy to see why a patient in coma must count on the nurse for everything that is required by the problem. It is not so easy to understand what is meant when a patient makes insistent demands on nurses but is able to get out of bed. It is more difficult to understand why a patient suffering coronary occlusion insists on taking care of himself. These are persisting difficulties in situations in which a nurse can help the patient to develop his personality by facing a difficulty together.

Personality formation in infancy: background information

In order to understand her own personality and that of the patient, as they interact in nursing situations, it is necessary for the professional nurse to appreciate the dynamic interaction that occurs in early infancy and childhood, as personality is undergoing formation.

Every infant is born having certain "raw materials" from which personality is formed. Briefly, these include: (1) a physique and its capacity for developing a pattern of movement; (2) a capacity for expressing temperament including rate, rhythm, and depth of the ability to perceive and to feel; (3) a capacity for reaching and functioning at a level of intelligence.[1]

[1] Harold Rugg, *Foundations for American Education* (New York, World Book Company, 1947), p. 169. A useful summarizing discussion of the "psychology of personality" is given on pages 169-205.

Every infant is also born into a culture having forces upon which it is dependent for survival. Although *the biology of an infant unfolds itself and organizes according to its perception of experience,* it seems self-evident that the human organism would die if external conditions essential to its growing were left entirely to chance. There are already existing forces outside the organism and in the context of culture into which it is born that are required for life to continue. It is the *interaction of cultural forces with the characteristic expression of a particular infant's biological constitution that determines personality.* Cultural forces are expressed and exemplified by the adults who provide essential conditions and from whom the infant acquires the existing mores, customs, and beliefs of a given culture.

Enough is not yet known concerning personality formation in order to assert that whatever the constitutional make-up at birth, a productive personality can be formed. So-called faulty constitutional make-up for whatever reason —genetic, uterine default, chemical imbalance—provide serious challenges for students of personality. It can be inferred that the shaping of personality from "raw materials," which constitutes the creative role of motherhood, is always hampered by limiting factors existing in the personality and outside awareness of the mother or her surrogate. It can be inferred that the awaiting culture manifests other limiting factors: an economic situation in a family that demands that a philosophy of scarcity or of plenty intrudes itself into the life of that family; an intellectual climate that demands a philosophy of inquiry and first-hand experiencing *or* one that demands rote learning and conforming to others leading to quick formation of habits. These limiting factors, and many others that might be cited, influence a particular infant during its formative years and affect the personality that is formed.

Whatever is present in the constitutional make-up of an infant at birth is expressed in a family or cultural situation. Adults respond to the infant's expression of his biology in ways that are rewarding or punishing to the infant. An infant who awakens often and cries lustily for food is expressing its biology; the infant who is quiet, sleeps long periods, and must often be awakened for feeding is also expressing its constitutional make-up. Whether the mother of these two infants *wants* two active ones or two quiet babies makes a difference to the one who is not accepted *as he is*. The kinds of responses a representative of a cultural group makes to the infant's natural expression of constitutional endowment permits or limits maximum unfolding of potential capacities. It is in the dynamic interaction—an infant who is completely helpless participating in an ongoing family—that personality is structured and the basic forms of its expression determined.

Each infant and child need a flexible pattern within which his biological constitution can find full expression, as it organizes itself slowly along ever more productive lines. Providing an environment in which self-directed expression can unfold is a difficult creative task. It requires knowledge and appreciation of developmental phases undergone by the infant, social requirements and their effects on the learning process operating within the child, and the psychological tasks that each infant and child faces as growing up takes place. Faith in the ability of a human being to organize himself is in direct opposition to the notion that a child is something to be "licked into shape," quickly and with dispatch. It requires recognition by all adults relating to infants and children that those forces within themselves that cry out, compulsively demanding that the child be limited in its expression to behavior that brings cultural approbation, are the very forces that are most often not understood. Yet, taking responsibility for the formation of personality in others requires understanding of personal needs, demands, and expectations that operate to distort interpersonal relations and to limit the growth of others.

Personality has been variously defined: Sullivan refers to it as a pattern that is relatively stable and that characterizes persisting situations in the life of an individual.[2] May defines it in terms of "social stimulus value"; that is, in describing the personality of others we describe the impression he makes or the way he influences others, rather than his reactions to situations.[3] Guthrie defines personality in terms of "habit adjustment," as the actions of a given individual in a given situation in response to various cues.[4] Watson defined personality as the total assets and liabilities that determine an individual's action.[5]

Fromm makes a distinction between "character structure" and personality.[6] Character represents the core or basic orientations toward life as they are learned and imbedded into the functional structure of an individual and expressed in personality. Character structure is the governing base from which personality makes its selective responses on the level of behavior. Whatever term seems more useful to nursing will be selected; however, when nurses wish to provide experiences with patients that aid them in expanding their personality and its functioning it is necessary for each nurse to examine her basic orientations toward life and their relation to present attitudes expressed in behavior and in relations with people.

The infant's biological functioning and the need for acculturation set up certain requirements, or *psychological tasks,* which every infant and child must undergo with relative success in order to develop a sound basis for mature functioning of personality as an adult. It is the degree of success with which each of these tasks is undergone that de-

[2] H. S. Sullivan, *The Meaning of Anxiety in Psychiatry and in Life* (Washington, D.C., William Alanson White Psychiatric Foundation), pamphlet, p. 50.

[3] P. S. Schilles, *Psychology at Work* (New York, Whittlesey House, 1932), paper by Mark May, "The Foundations of Personality," pp. 81-101.

[4] J. McV. Hunt (ed.), *Personality and the Behavior Disorders* (New York, The Ronald Cross Company, 1944), Vol. I, Ch. 2, Edwin R. Guthrie, "Personality in terms of associative learning."

[5] J. B. Watson, *The New Behaviorism* (New York, W. W. Norton & Company, 1930), p. 304.

[6] Erich Fromm, *Escape from Freedom* (New York, Farrar & Rinehart, Inc., 1941), p. 278.

termines the basic orientations toward life that an individual will later express in all situations in life in which he participates. The outcome is his base line in learning to live with people.

The tasks of growing up have been considered in various forms, such as "developmental tasks," "building blocks of personality," "psychosexual stages of personality organization," and the like.[7, 8, 9] In this text we are referring only to psychological tasks that are required of infants and children. When they are successfully learned at each era of development, biological capacities are used productively and relations with people lead to productive living. When they are not successfully learned they carry over into adulthood and attempts at learning continue in devious ways, more or less impeded by conventional adaptations that provide a superstructure over the base line of actual learning. Psychological tasks have to do with total experiences during a particular era and subsequent stages in development. During one era they may be more or less specifically focused on particular bodily areas but the learning situation is more general and often takes in other areas of the body to express what has been experienced earlier in relations with people.

Interactive experiences that affect the formation of personality in early childhood are general and include the communication of attitudes, feelings, and ideas expressed by parents and surrogates to children. However, psychoanalytic literature is abundant in showing how these interactive experiences also cluster about oral, anal, and genital pleasures and functions as they are experienced and integrated into total bodily functioning during early years of life. The phys-

[7] Robert J. Havighurst, *Developmental Tasks and Education* (Chicago. The University of Chicago Press, 1948), pamphlet.

[8] Sigmund Freud, *Basic Writings* (New York, Random House, Inc., Modern Library Edition, 1938). See also: O. Spurgeon English and Gerald H. J. Pearson, *Common Neuroses of Children and Adults* (New York, W. W. Norton & Company, 1937), especially pp. 1-83.

[9] J. D. Brown, *Psychodynamics of Abnormal Behavior* (New York, McGraw-Hill Book Company, Inc., 1940), sec. III, pp. 162-68.

iological functioning of these bodily areas is such that the *culture,* in its impact upon the child and in ways that adults aid it to acquire customs with regard to food and food habits, toilet training, and sexual behavior, *readily invades and distorts physiological functioning.* Various degrees of anxiety are generated and then become localized in these bodily areas. When such invasion is in direct and continuous opposition to physiological expression and demands constitutional reorientation in terms of cultural wishes, these same zones of interaction become the field through which distortions of personality are expressed.

The oral, anal, and genital areas are perceived by the infant as aspects of the body that give pleasure and satisfy emergent needs; the discovery of each new outlet for satisfaction is a growth experience for the infant and child. When needs are deprived and the discovery of parts of the body is prohibited the anxiety of the parent is communicated to the infant, as disapproval, and the child adapts by using less natural behavior in order to achieve approval in lieu of satisfaction, as a way of maintaining feelings of security.

The more important factor when culture invades infant physiology in a traumatic way is not that the child adapts by taking on behavior approved by the culture, for this is the eventual aim of all relations between mother and child. It is that the interpersonal relations are distorted in terms of the child merely maintaining comfort while learning is seriously interfered with, so that the child distorts the meaning of events and later resymbolizes and synthesizes them in terms of feelings that are not formulated or understood. An example may clarify what is meant:

A four-year-old child is greatly disturbed by a physical disability which her mother is undergoing at a particular time. The child shows no regard for the fact that her mother is experiencing pain in her leg or that she cannot bend over to pick things up or take long walks. Yet the child, to a greater degree than ever before, insists on dropping things, demands that her mother pick them up, whacks her mother on the leg, and begs to be taken on long walks. The child's actions can be understood as an appropriate response to her fear that her mother is falling apart, and will not be available to take care of her. The mother can understand and respect these feelings or she can moralize and demand that the child show her some consideration—which in effect requires that the child will not express and therefore will be unable to identify her real feelings. With moralizing, then, the child is asked to distort the meaning of what is happening to her and to her mother, and in order to continue to have support, acceptance, and approval she must adapt her behavior in direct opposition to her own feelings. She can do this by resymbolizing her role; where she was allowed to be a child she could live the role of a child but this role can be resymbolized so that she takes on the role of mother, giving unconditional care to her mother instead of expecting such care as the rightful expectation of any child. This changes the relationship of mother and child.

Distorted meanings of events, and acquired behavior that is based upon a discrepancy between feelings and actions appropriate to those feelings, carry over as basic ways of looking at one's self and at life; they enter into all later life situations in which it is the feelings—never fully understood in their relations to past events—rather than the events themselves that are re-enacted in new situations such as in nursing. Therefore, the growing child and later the adult, under these conditions, tends to view all new situations in terms of older feelings of deprivation and dissatisfaction, rather than considering them as new ones having merit on their own. Behavior acceptable to the culture, when it is an adaptation that is forced prematurely by adult coercions before the meaning is clearly understood by an individual, tends to generate feelings that are inacceptable to the self.

"Habit formations" associated with oral, anal, and genital areas consist in more than accepting culturally approved ways to eat, to defecate, and to have sexual experience. They provide focal points for dramatizing unmet needs and for experiencing and integrating new relationships in subsequent situations, long after the habits are in operation and with seemingly little connection to them. Infant-feeding patterns, toilet-training practices, attitudes toward sexual activities are communicated to infants and children and provide foci for undergoing important psychological tasks in learning that speed up or limit the use of constitutional endowment of an individual.

Psychological tasks, considered as psychodynamically important learning experiences, are constants in the life of every infant and child. They are interpersonal experiences that must be undergone with maximum success if sound foundations for health are to be laid. Observations made at later periods in life will show the soundess of earlier learning, or the shakiness of the conventional superstructure that has been substituted for learning. The timing, the intensity, the strength of individual expression in each task are functions of varying constitutional factors, which also demand expression as the tasks are undergone. They are influenced by the needs, hopes, beliefs, and expectations of adults who are relating to a particular individual or child. Each task represents an inescapable experience necessary for learning to live with people, undergone when the young normally undergo feelings of powerlessness, helplessness, and of inability to defend themselves physically against power greater than that they themselves feel. The manner of undergoing psychological tasks prepares well or ill for meeting challenges to psychobiological functioning in adulthood; each task is always experienced in terms of both inner and outer demands and leaves the individual with ways of looking at his world and at the recurring difficulties that he will face during his future life.

The first psychological task: learning to count on others

A newborn infant is only capable of feeling *comfort and discomfort*. As the infant grows these two feelings are differentiated further, such as comfort in being warm, having a full stomach, and the like. Experiencing the discomfort of pain, deprivation of a need, or of being alone are also differentiations that come later as the meaning of the first whole impression of comfort or discomfort are more clearly understood. A newborn infant cannot differentiate himself from his mother at once; he knows by way of his feelings that discomfort is relieved and that comfort is felt but does not yet associate the satisfaction of needs with the functions of someone outside himself; he experiences the comfort, the discomfort, and the relief of discomfort as a unit—a series of momentary states that make up a whole but unclear experience.

From birth the infant is able to communicate to others that discomfort is felt, and he uses the *cry as his tool* for letting adults know about his uncomfortable state. Gradually the infant begins to recognize that there is a relationship between using the cry and restoration of feelings of comfort. Where comfort was restored earlier in some unknown way the infant now begins to perceive that when he cries something large comes toward him and *a satisfaction-response* soon follows as comfort is restored. This sequence of events might be thought of as the first recognition that through his own efforts, by crying and making his discomfort known, he can again gain a feeling of satisfaction. As this experience is differentiated further, as the infant becomes more and more able to be aware of his surroundings, he comes to recognize that the something large is always the same—and thus he learns that he is dependent upon his mother or her surrogate for achieving a feeling of satisfaction or comfort.

The earlier psychologists misinterpreted what was going on in the mother and child relationship as it is described above. They felt that the child learned to cry for attention and that giving it laid down a pattern of behavior in which the child would always cry in order to get attention. More recent points of view show that the infant uses the tools for communication that are available to him, and that he uses them until other tools supplant them in achieving satisfaction of wants and wishes, in achieving a feeling of comfort. They show further that permitting the infant's natural tools to operate leads more readily to the development of other more culturally approved ones than does deprivation of infant needs at this time.

So far we have described three important observations of the infant: the feeling of discomfort, the communication of it through his own efforts and by crying, and the achievement of a satisfaction response when discomfort is relieved. The feelings of discomfort referred to includes being hungry, wet, cold, etc. When the mother responds warmly and unconditionally to these needs felt by the child she also experiences a satisfaction response, in that her motherly functions have been carried out. There is a mutuality about the satisfaction response, and the concomitant feelings of comfort are communicated interpersonally from mother to child. If, however, the mother cannot respond warmly and feels anxious about the care of her child, her anxiety is communicated to the infant as a new kind of discomfort that is empathized by the infant. *Empathic observation* is also a tool in infancy by which felt-relations in the mother-child situation are observed though not understood by the infant.

When a mother appreciates that feelings are communicated between the infant and herself, and when she can respond in an unconditional way to the infant expressing his needs in terms of the rate, rhythm, and depth of feeling that are inherent in his biological make-up, *the infant gradually learns that he can count on his mother for help, with good feeling, when he needs it.* The infant's dependence upon his mother is not discriminated at first, but he needs to learn that he is separable from her and that he is dependent upon others; dependency must be learned and accepted in a clear and comfortable way.

Dependence upon others is at first known as a felt-relation. That is, it is not known as an intellectual operation or reasoning but by way of feelings.[10] An infant develops a sense of power and a feeling that his own efforts, as expressed in the cry, lead him to feel satisfaction. The wish to struggle and to make wants and needs known is later expressed in other vocal behavior—such as asking for help when it is needed. This extension of feelings of power in vocal behavior is possible only when the cry of the infant is heeded and thus respected as a tool of self-expression.

The infant learns from experience with his mother that his wants are valid and that his efforts to communicate them are respected. This learning occurs when the mother can make unconditional love available to the infant. By unconditional love is meant the prompt response to the child's communication that he feels discomfort. Love is conditional when a mother's attitude communicates, "I will love you if you are quiet," "if you do not disturb me," or "if you will do exactly as I say, namely, wait for your food until I am ready and eat all of it when I give it to you." Conditional love is oriented to the needs and the program of work of the mother; unconditional love is governed by the needs and demands of the infant. Every infant requires unconditional attention at first. When it is given the infant can develop a full-fledged wish to sharpen his tools of communication and to struggle with the object world and in his own terms to master it. These are all first steps to wishes that emerge later and ones that are subject to greater social approval.

The wish to struggle in order to achieve satisfaction of wants is reinforced and leads to "positive groping" or forward

---

[10] A fuller knowledge of all that is involved in this experience is well documented in: Benjamin Spock and Mabel Huschka, *The Psychological Aspects of Pediatric Practice,* reprinted by courtesy of Appleton-Century-Crofts, Inc., and made available through the New York State Committee on Mental Hygiene of the State Charities Aid Association, 1938, uses the terms "positive groping" and "negative withdrawal" in a very helpful discussion of infant behavior patterns. H. S. Sullivan, *Conceptions of Modern Psychiatry* (Washington, D.C., William Alanson White Psychiatric Foundation, 1947), pp. 14-42 for a discussion of the evolution of personality in infancy. Hunt, *op. cit.,* pp. 621-51, paper by Margaret A. Ribble, "Infantile experience in relation to personality development."

movement in becoming socialized. This wish extinguishes easily under conditions that produce anxiety in the child —such as communication of dissatisfaction with the child through the mother's attitudes, voice tones, method of handling the infant, and the like. The mother's goals, when care that she offers is conditional, function as barriers to the achievement of the infant's goal, namely, comfort or satisfaction. The infant's mind and his nervous system are not yet sufficiently developed, nor does he have tools of communication that go beyond his immediate feelings, that can be used to deal with more complex tasks in living. "Negative withdrawal" is a response that is an adaptation in very young infants when needs are not met promptly and when feelings of satisfaction and comfort are denied in a continuing way. The infant gives up the struggle for the satisfaction response and the goal connected with it. This phenomenon may be observed in any newborn nursery where infants are permitted to cry until time for feeding, according to a schedule. The infant expends the energy crying and finally "knocks himself out" and can be aroused at feeding time only with great difficulty. This behavior is no different from extreme degrees of withdrawal seen in psychiatric patients, when ongoing needs have been deprived year after year and where a solution to the problem has been achieved by giving up, permanently, all activities that express and achieve satisfaction of wants.

Self-reliance in the infant is expressed in terms of relying upon the tools of communication that are available to him. The importance of the cry has already been discussed. The infant also empathizes what is felt about him, as it is communicated through the kind of handling that he receives. Empathy refers to an ability to feel what is going on in a situation without specifically being able to discuss and to identify elements of it in awareness. The infant feels what others feel as they relate to him. If their attitudes reward his crying as a struggle or effort to express what is wanted, and if they communicate that they share in the satisfaction that the infant feels when discomfort is relieved, the infant then "knows" that his efforts are respected for what they are. If on the other hand anxiety is communicated through attitudes and handling that express dissatisfaction with the infant's crying, the way he feeds, the amount that is taken, the restlessness that he shows, the infant again "knows" that others do not appreciate his efforts or share in his feelings of satisfaction.

Passive receptivity is thought to be a characteristic of infant behavior. The infant actively takes in, swallows, and absorbs what is offered to him. The ability to take in food is usually highlighted in discussions about infant behavior but the infant also takes into himself the attitudes of others around him. He has no attitudes of his own; he has only the capacity to feel comfort and discomfort and to struggle to make his wants known in order to feel satisfaction. The infant takes on the attitudes of those around him. If they permit him to have his own wants, to struggle to express them, and to achieve satisfaction in response to them he slowly becomes aware that his wants can be communicated and that others reward his efforts in ways that bring satisfaction. That is, *he learns in a clear and comfortable way that he is dependent upon others for the achievement of his wishes.* Thus, he begins to differentiate himself from others and to count on them for help when it is needed.

When an infant is not rewarded for expressing his ability to communicate that he has wants, and when his goal of satisfaction is not readily achieved through others, the infant's passive receptivity is reinforced. The infant's capacity to differentiate himself from others is arrested, since his helplessness is reinforced when the tools at his disposal are not respected. As in any other frustration, the infant can vary his goal in the light of experience, but he must do so on the basis of feelings only since intellectual operations are not yet possible for him. The infant can give up the goal, namely, the wish to struggle to express what is wanted in order to feel satisfaction. Or, "negative withdrawal" may be reinforced as a fixed response. The identification of wants and the periods during which they will or will not be satisfied is left to the designation of others. It is difficult to separate from a mother upon whom one is wholly dependent for identifying and for fulfilling wants. When an infant must wait until someone else gives him what is thought to be needed, he becomes less able to identify and to communicate what is wanted and thus is also less able to differentiate himself from his mother.[11]

When an infant is not aided to differentiate himself from others and to recognize his wants, as well as to struggle to communicate them to others, an insatiable dependency longing develops. For purposes of clarity in discussion, it is well to differentiate dependence and a longing for dependency. Dependence is recognized through experience with a world that is satisfying and sustaining and a world in which one participates. Dependency longings derive from perception of a world that is threatening and hostile, one that does not permit struggle to express wants and needs, and one in which all of the effort expended comes through others. Dependence is a consequence of experiencing freedom of expression and choice, even in when to feed and to be comfortable in an infant; it requires a permissive world where freedom to express wants and differences in rate, rhythm, and depth of feeling is allowed even on a trial and error basis. Dependency longings, on the other hand, are learned through interpersonal relations with people who demand, deny, withhold, barter, or gratify in order to get conformity to their goals and patterns of what is desirable behavior.[12]

Longings for dependency develop when a mother rejects or overprotects her infant.[13] An infant experiences rejection when his wants are completely denied. His wants are simple; they include the feeling of comfort that goes with being held closely in welcoming arms of the mother, a full stomach, comfortable clothing, and a bed. He feels rejection when his

[11] Fromm, *op. cit.,* pp. 22-23.
[12] *Ibid.*
[13] Karen Horney, *New Ways in Psychoanalysis* (New York, W. W. Norton & Company, 1939), pp. 74-75. Defines "basic anxiety" as an outcome of these experiences.

mother's arms are not forthcoming, when he is discomforted, or when he is feeding as when a bottle is propped in his bed. The infant's wish to struggle and to communicate his wants is also smothered when a rejecting mother overcompensates for her genuine feelings about the infant by being overconcerned about his welfare. The infant will be disturbed during sleep or feeding if the mother too often makes sure that he is all right. The mother will show overconcern about the amount of milk that is taken and feel sure that the infant should have more. The infant's right to determine how much it can take at a particular feeding is not seen in perspective of what is taken during a whole day; each feeding time becomes an opportunity to show anxiety and concern about the infant's welfare as a way of demonstrating what is thought to be genuine mother love.

A mother who cares for her infant, wants it to, is genuinely concerned that it will grow and develop and become a productive person, will at the same time have faith in her capacity to show her interest in a helpful way. She will enjoy her infant and permit it to enjoy closeness with her. She will recognize its way of expressing needs and she will respond knowing that the infant is learning to respect her as a person who offers help when it is needed. She will not intrude on the infant's comfort to satisfy her own urges to hold and to fondle the baby.

Dependence and dependency longings as seen in nursing

Dependence upon others for help when needed requires ability to identify what is wanted, to struggle to communicate wishes to others, and to feel free to make use of assistance that is offered in solving a personal problem—such as medical illness. *A longing for dependency* operates as an insatiable need in an individual who either takes it for granted that others will know what is needed, without any intervening communication from the individual to the person providing help, or who denies that help of any kind will ever be useful. Both ways of expressing a longing for dependency were found to be useful in earlier situations in life in which the individual was not fully respected as one who could make known his wants and struggle toward their achievement with the help of other persons.

In nursing situations both dependence and degrees of dependency longings operate in patients. They require different degrees of "mothering" as a component in nursing. Several experiences documented by nurses illustrate ways in which nurses face the psychological task with patients who have not yet learned that dependence is a necessary component in interdependent relations with people.

A patient came to the hospital for herniorrhaphy and in the operating room a nurse was asked to hold him in position for a spinal injection. She noticed that the patient's knees were trembling and that he kept opening and closing his hands. When she held his hands during the procedure the trembling stopped and the patient appeared less upset about what was happening to him. After the anesthesia was given the patient's position was changed and the nurse prepared to leave in order to go about her other duties in the operating room. The following conversation took place.

Patient:	*Nurse:*
"Please don't leave me nurse. Stay with me, and hold my hand. If you leave me alone I just know that I'll be a sissy. I'm afraid."	The nurse checked with the scrub nurse who said it was all right to stay. She permitted the patient to hold her hand and listened while he talked occasionally about the operation in progress.
(When the operation was over the patient said:) "Oh, thank you nurse. I wouldn't have survived except for your help."	Having met the patient's need for feeling close to someone as he was undergoing surgery relieved his tension and made it possible for him to recognize that others will help when help is needed.

A second experience in the operating room shows how nearness of the nurse and skillful listening can aid the patient to clarify some of his feelings related to a longing for dependency.

Patient:

"I have heard that Dr. Jones is a very good surgeon and that he can make me better. You know, I can't hear from my left ear, and I can't see very well. I wish I could hear again after this operation."

"Nurse, am I boring you? I know it is hard to understand me, but I can talk better with only one person instead of a group of people."

"Oh, that's nice of you to say that. Nobody has ever said that to me. In the other building everyone was against me."

"Yes, I guess it's because they couldn't understand me. I tried to be friendly with them, but you know I can't hear well and they are all against me."

"They are all against me because I am a Jew."

Nurse:

After this remark the nurse was called away but explained that she would come back, since it seemed the patient wanted her to stay with him.

"You are not boring me. I have been able to understand all that you have said to me."

"Everyone was against you?"

"They are all against you because you can't hear well?"

In the above experience the patient used a roundabout way to communicate his dependence upon the nurse. There is not enough evidence to know whether a longing for dependence is expressed or not but when the nurse met his need, the patient could express his real feelings about why his need to belong was not met by other patients in his ward. In this experience the nurse at first tried to reassure the patient by pointing out that she could understand him. However, when he then revealed hostile feelings toward others she realized that further reassurance wouldn't be of any use to the patient, and so she reflected back what had been said. The nurse was surprised to find out that the patient would uncover his real feelings so quickly. However, he was about to undergo an operation and had considerable anxiety about taking anesthesia and in this instance the nurse aided him to use the energy derived from the anxiety or tension to examine his feelings. He was able to bring out into the open what he considered the reason why he could not depend upon others to be friendly with him.

A third experience illustrates another variation of longing for dependency. A patient admitted to a medical ward, with a diagnosis of coronary occlusion, remained about two hours and then got out of bed, put on his bathrobe and slippers, walked out of the hospital and drove home. He had been dissatisfied with his accommodations, angry that the doctor had sent him to the hospital in the first place, and upset because his tray was not served to him immediately. He took it for granted that the hospital staff would know at once what was needed and that they would respond to his needs without further communication from him. His wife sat patiently beside him and said nothing, then walked out quietly beside him as he left the hospital.

The nurses had not served his tray because the doctor had not ordered one in advance and it was necessary to call to the diet kitchen and to wait until the tray was brought up. When nurses make observations in experiences with patients suffering coronary disease they often generalize that many of them have deep longings for dependency that are overcompensated for in work activities. Acting on this generalization in situations with other new patients the nurse would offer unconditional attention in the form of her presence, until the tray could be brought in. This relationship could develop further as time went on, so that the patient could gain some interest in interdependent relations with nurses. Most coronary occlusions are observed in patients who cannot express dependence or interdependence and who are unaware of the longing for dependency that has been covered up in their excessive drive to have things their own way, to run a business and to make money at the expense of the needs of their employees.

A fourth experience illustrates the problems connected with dependence and longings for it.

A patient came to the hospital suffering mucous colitis and was taken to the operating room for the first stage operation. He refused the spinal anesthesia. His father, a doctor, came over and patted his hand saying, "Now, let the doctor give you this medicine. It will relieve your discomfort and get you ready for the operation." The boy complied. Soon the father left the room and once again the patient remonstrated against treatment, saying, "The surgeon is trying to kill me." He appeared very frightened.

In this experience we can see complete dependence upon someone else to interpret what is needed and what this need will do for the problem. Compliant behavior occurred in response to a parental command but when the parent was not present the patient again felt free to raise objections to what was going on in the situation and identify his interpretation of events. This patient was not aware of his need to rebel against dependence upon others, nor had he been aided to identify his wishes and goals in behalf of his medical problem. The surgeon's efforts were viewed as an interference that threatened life and show that he cannot afford to depend upon what others will do even though they promise that it will make him well.

A fifth experience shows how nurses can cope with longings for dependence. A patient was hospitalized for peptic ulcer several times a year for a few years in succession. He distrusted nurses who brought in medications or milk every two hours and always questioned their value. He would frequently ring five or ten minutes before his treatments were due and remind nurses not to get too busy and thus overlook his medicines. He criticized doctors and nurses alike and in general found fault with what was offered to him. The nurses on that particular floor decided to select one nurse who would make it her business to drop in well in advance of medication or feeding time. The nurse would listen to his comments without offering any advice or reassurance. She would then announce that it was almost time for his milk or his medicine and that she would bring it in at once. Nurses took turns for two week periods and it took about six weeks before the patient learned that he could count on the nurses for the attention that he needed. 'His relations with nurses improved accordingly and he has not been hospitalized since.

Nurses have two responsibilities in their relations with patients who express longings for dependence: (1) to help the patient to learn that nurses can be counted on for help when needed; this learning occurs through demonstrated interest as illustrated in the experience described above; (2) to aid the patient to become aware of his wants and to improve his ways of expressing what those wants are. Patients who can identify their needs do not present serious difficulties to nurses. Patients who are overly receptive, accepting everything that is done for them as remarkable and asking nothing of nurses, and those who insist on doing everthing for themselves even when critically ill, do require skillful nursing in order that they may learn to recognize what their needs and wants are and how they may best be met in the present situation.

Passive receptivity is illustrated in the following experience. Mr. Smith was admitted to the hospital with a diagnosis of carcinoma of the larynx for which a total laryngectomy was done. The patient required a permanent tracheotomy tube in his throat as a result. It can be seen that his surgical problem falls in the oral area and thus reawakens feelings connected with the oral stage of psychosexual development. There is no evidence on how the patient was prepared psychologically for this operation, but after it he became completely helpless and dependent upon nurses. Some nurses expressed their opinions as, "he is unco-operative," "he acts like a baby," or "he refuses to do anything for himself." The patient was allowed bathroom privileges but "refused to get up." Some nurses felt that the patient was "trying to get attention."

When the nature of the difficulty is examined closely it can be seen that this patient is forced back upon infantile ways of making known what his wants are; he could not speak and so ordinary communication was cut off for him. Perhaps he could have written down what he wanted but this was not tried. When a patient "acts like a baby" and "refuses to take care of himself" it seems pretty evident that psychologically he is incapable of so doing and that he needs to have someone else do what is needed. If nurses in this instance had willingly given him unconditional care, they could also have observed his responses and made interpretations with him that might have been useful: "You feel that you need me to give you a bath," "You feel pretty helpless without being able to speak," or, "I will leave some paper and a pencil here and perhaps you will want to write down some of the things you want that I have not noticed."

Some nurses feel that "catering" to the patient in this way keeps him a baby, but the principle that operates for infants and adults is as follows: *When emergent needs are met more mature needs emerge.* Mothering a patient who needs "mothering" makes it possible for that patient to grow and to become independent of a mother surrogate, as a give and take, person to person relationship develops. Denying this patient the kind of nursing indicated by his expression of needs, through his behavior, is a way of making it impossible for him to feel satisfaction of wants that he cannot communicate. The patient must then redouble his efforts to show that he needs help, and it is evident in the data presented that this is what the patient did—he became more helpless, more powerless, and more unable to reach the goals of others until his wants were satisfied. His behavior may be viewed as a way of trying to feel safe, trying to make sure that others will see what is needed. It is a way of attempting to restore communication, of getting close to people with whom he feels he has been "cut off," since he cannot tell them how he feels.

An experience documented by a nurse illustrates the difficulty encountered when patients deny that they need help of any kind. The patient was a business woman who had been unusually active and independent in her work, and then suffered hemiplegia. She resented being waited on and found it most unrewarding to be told that she should do certain exercises that would restore the function in her affected arm. The nurse first established a relationship with the patient, paying as little attention to the exercises as she could in view of written directives. As the nurse and patient came to know and to respect one another the patient revealed that she was an antique dealer and that she had been planning to put antique buttons on cards for an exhibit that was to be held at a much later date. The nurse seized upon this interest and helped the patient to set this as her goal, and together they outlined activities that would be required for reaching it. First the patient was willing to hold a sponge in her hand and to squeeze it until her hand gained some strength. Then a pencil was inserted in the sponge and writing was started. The patient kept her buttons handy and soon she was ready to start putting them on cards. With her energy channelized in the activities directed toward her own goal she became less hostile toward her family, and as she found herself being able to do things for herself she would do them, mentioning to the nurse, "I can do that myself." In other words, through a dependent relationship with the nurse she was able to recognize her need and to use the help made available to her and gradually to put it aside, as the nurse responded to cues that indicated that she could successfully take care of herself.

Sometimes patients will expect and accept full nursing care as a way of making up for full denial of ordinary needs for dependence on others in their home. For example, Mr. Light was hospitalized for ten days for a herniorrhaphy. According to early ambulation, he was allowed out of bed the next day. However, he retained private duty nurses for his entire hospital stay. He insisted that he needed help because he was "too weak." Nevertheless, he carried on long conversations, read the daily papers, and later on walked around quite a bit. When his wife visited him it could be observed that she looked to him for all decisions, that she was most dependent upon him for approval and direction. The patient's illness seemed to afford him an opportunity to sample what it felt like to be taken care of without sacrificing his prestige as an important and successful businessman. The nurses helped the patient as he desired, saying, "It is nice to have someone help you to take a bath and a shave, even though you are able to do it yourself." The patient was fully aware of his present feelings and was merely using his operation as an opportunity to restore himself for his usual role in which there seemed to be little room for dependence on others.

Another patient, age thirteen, who entered the hospital for a triple arthrodesis, showed unusually strong longings for dependency following anesthesia. She cried a great deal and called for her mother. She asserted that she couldn't turn herself onto her side without help, although actually she should have been able to do so. When the patient wanted a drink of water she called for a nurse to help her, rather than reaching over to her bedside table for the glass of water. When she couldn't think of specific things to ask for she again would cry for her mother. When the nurses carried out her requests she would stop crying.

A number of courses of action are open to nurses in this situation. Recognizing that the age of the patient means that she is approaching the adolescent dilemma of working through her need for dependence and for independence in her relations with her mother, the nurses might feel that they *should make* her more self-reliant, demanding that she do things for herself. However, when needs for dependence are deprived they go underground and operate as a longing that makes it more impossible for feelings of interdependence to generate. The nurses could respond to the needs of the patient and help her to identify her feelings about her operation, and how it has made her feel and think of herself as a person. They might sit with her when she cries and, while permitting full expression of the wish to cry, give the patient the support of the nurse's presence. Most likely the patient would put aside crying as a tool of communication and begin to use speech, letting the nurses know why she feels she wants to cry. Other nurses might tell the patient to stop crying, "There is nothing to cry about, after all, the operation is over and the doctor did a good job." This is a way of letting the patient know that you cannot accept her as she is; that the patient will be accepted *if* she stops crying, *if* she does things for herself, *if* she makes no demands upon nurses. The patient must deny her own feelings and needs in order to be accepted and liked by a nurse who is *conditional* in her relations with the patient.

In order to decide on the actions a nurse might take when patients express dependence or longings for dependence, it is necessary to look at what learning is taking place. When needs and requests are denied, and the patient compelled to fend for himself, does the patient perceive that: *others do not like me; others do not want to help me; others say I must do things that I cannot do.* When needs are met does the patient learn: *others are willing to help me, therefore I must be someone they respect and like; others are willing to help me and perhaps I can help them too, I will try; when you are sick nurses are so helpful.*

There is a great deal of social learning that takes place in a situation where nursing is offered. The patient learns more about people and what they think of him through their attitudes toward him than he does about medical information. A patient cannot take in new information unless there is a warm relationship between patient and nurse in which each has come to know and to respect the wishes of the other. A warm relationship begins to develop when nurses meet the needs of patients in ways that permit the patient to become aware of what those needs are. Often after an illness the thing that stands out in sharpest focus in the patient's mind is the attitudes of the nurse toward him when he felt dependent upon nursing for help.

Summary

Patients need to learn to count on nurses for comfort and satisfaction of their wants in much the same manner that infants learn to achieve satisfaction through their mothers. Very young infants can only use their ability to cry to communicate their discomfort to others. Patients often cry for the same reason, or they may express their needs for "mothering" through behavior that indicates helplessness, powerlessness, and inability to act in their own behalf in making wants known. Failure to permit the patient to receive nursing when he feels helpless is a way of demanding that feelings of helplessness be dissociated from awareness. Responding to the patient's expression of helplessness is a way of helping the patient to achieve satisfaction of needs so that more mature ones can emerge. The patient's behavior is a way of struggling to communicate his feelings and wants that cannot be communicated in a forthright verbal manner. Assisting the patient to get all of the help that he needs and at the same time aiding him to explore his feelings and to identify his wants is a way of helping the patient to mature. A relationship that demonstrates warmth and acceptance of the patient *as he is* restores the patient's faith in himself and makes it possible for him to identify with others and to take on attitudes of helpfulness toward others, as he learns them from nurses who help him. A nurse needs to be clear about how she feels about giving help to patients when she believes they are capable of doing more than their behavior indicates. The nurse's view of the patient, and the goals that she sets for him, act as interferences or barriers to the patient's goal— to be mothered during a crisis that makes him feel powerless. Aggressive behavior in response to the frustration felt by the patient, when his goals are denied, usually takes the form of refusal to comply with nurses, redoubling demands for help, or apathy. Each patient a nurse aids to work through his feelings of dependence or his longings for mothering that have been denied in the past becomes a member of society who can identify what he wants and who can struggle toward the achievement of those wants. When the patient has been enabled to feel that he does not have to struggle alone, that help when needed is forthcoming, he tends more to identify wants that are socially approved and that are good for others as well as for himself.

Dependence is a recurring problem in nursing. The way in which it is met is determined by the learning that nurses want to have take place in patients. This learning is more likely to be social learning, about people, about their interactive relations, than it is information about a medical problem. Information is useful when it is given in an interpersonal relation felt to be warm, accepting, and relatively comfortable—a relationship in which the patient can be himself, can have his own feelings, and can express them, knowing that nurses will not make judgments and not disapprove.

CHAPTER 9

Learning to Delay Satisfaction

Overview

IN NURSING SITUATIONS it is not always possible to grant patients full expression of all their wants or wishes and still meet the requirements of a treatment plan outlined by a professional team. It is often necessary to aid the patient in delaying his expected satisfactions, in varying his goals in the light of the reality of his medical problem. In order to know how patients can best be aided to learn to delay satisfaction of their wants, and to correlate this learning with the first psychological task, namely, learning to count on others for help when it is needed, as discussed in Chapter Eight, it is necessary to look at the period of personality formation most closely connected with the original learning of delay. The purpose of this chapter is to identify relationships between early childhood experiences with toilet training and personality formation and between cultural ways of interfering with wishes and wants and the carry-over in feelings that often operates in a medical problem. When nurses are faced with the task of helping a patient to delay his wants and wishes, and feelings of satisfaction connected with them, they need to understand these relationships to practice nursing intelligently.

189

Essential questions

What does a child learn during the period of toilet training? Who should decide when a child should learn socially approved bathroom habits. How does a child perceive the experience of learning to use a toilet? Can the experience be designed so that the child will want to learn to use a toilet in the same manner as adults? Is there a relationship between what is experienced during this period, by a child, and adult behavior in nursing situations? What are the recurring difficulties in relationships of nurse to patient that hark back to toilet training and to the mother and child relationship? What can a nurse do about it at this late date? These academically phrased questions are much the same as the problems faced by nurses when patients say: Why should I do it just because you or the doctor say so? Why should I give up eating candy just because I have diabetes; I don't like that diet you bring me anyway. Why should I stay in the hospital when my children need me at home? An examination of these questions and problems leads to understanding of some of the interpersonal difficulties that may not have been worked through in the mother and child, or subsequent relationships, and that seem to recur in situations in which nursing is required.

Personality formation in childhood: background information

Every individual must both experience and accept, with relatively good feeling, some interference with acquired ability to express wants, to produce, to decide, to formulate plans independently of others. Deference to the wishes of others often requires delaying satisfaction of one's own wishes; it is the first step in interdependent, social relations. The first learning experience, namely, learning to count on others for help when it is needed, lays the foundation for attitudes toward interferences to goals and wishes. During

childhood, adults and the culture generally begin to interfere with the direct expression of a child's wishes.[1] While this
is true in a general way, its implications can be seen more
specifically and sharply in considering the anal stage of psychosexual development that involves the period of toilet
training as defined by a family or a culture.

The physiological functioning of the very young child is
so geared that the body will act in its own best interest when
it is given an opportunity to do so. When the rectum is full
a young infant empties it at his convenience and thus feels
relief from discomfort. However, the growing child cannot
be permitted this freedom and consequently is expected to
adapt to the culturally approved ways—using the toilet as a
more acceptable place into which the feces in the rectum are
to be emptied. This is what society expects the child to be
able to do.

Some mothers wish their children to be toilet trained as
soon as possible, this being more convenient for the parent.
Other parents find it possible to be unconditional for a
longer period of time. In some cultures parents do not decide when the child will learn socially accepted practices but
leave it to the child to learn it from other children. Regardless of what age the parent decides upon to begin toilet
training, the child is not capable of taking on the social goal
until he has control of his sphincter muscles. For most children this is possible sometime during the second year.

During the period of toilet training the insecure mother,
who governs her behavior by what her neighbors or parents
expect of her rather than by what she feels is right for her
child, often feels the need to interfere too early with the
normal, natural bowel function of her child. She thinks of
it merely as a messy business and that toilet training will
cut down on the laundry that she has to do. However, the
child's ability to produce a stool is an emergent biological
activity rooted in the child; it is also a psychological experience that is felt as the ability to express productivity in his

[1] Weaning may be looked upon as an interference or frustration experience.

own right. The child becomes aware that he has produced this object through his own body. He is not bogged down with cultural attitudes about filth, and messiness, and germs, and consequently he perceives the stool according to its meaning for him. To him it means that he has delivered an interesting product from his own body and through his own efforts. If he has a warm dependent relationship with his mother he will offer it to her as a gift from him. This is the first step in the child's ability to give to others, since heretofore he has been getting or receiving from others. Because others have been giving things to him, he now feels that this valuable product is at last something of his own that he can give to others.

The child may also become very curious about this object of his own productivity. He will examine it, taste it, smear it, test it for consistency and hardness. He is fascinated about his product and wishes to find out what it is like.

Many mothers are unaware of the psychological experience that the child is undergoing in the foregoing activities, and that he is learning to explore the nature of the product of his personal power. Often they feel it "their duty," sometimes experienced as a compulsion, to force upon the child at once a standard of behavior that is ready-made, in advance of the wants and wishes of the child for socially approved behavior such as going to the bathroom to have a bowel movement that can be flushed down immediately, without further inquiry. Regardless of what kind of attitudes and methods the mother uses the child will adapt by conforming to accepted standards of behavior. But, when the mother uses rigorous training procedures and enforces rigid standards for toilet behavior, without permitting the child to complete the critical inquiry he makes into his product, she often requires that the events and the feelings connected with them be dissociated.

In psychiatric hospitals one can see many patients who smear feces day after day. Their records usually show that they were toilet trained very early, or that they were rendered powerless in many ways. Often there is no evidence of smearing, but this does not mean that it did not take place during childhood. It is more likely to mean that the parent has also dissociated the idea that her child could ever think of such a "dirty procedure."

The child is not weighed down by cultural attitudes of disgust about feces and so his curiosity can operate in its natural setting and in relation to whatever comes to his attention. However, when the attitude of disgust is communicated to the child by the parent, and the child quickly whisked off to the bathtub for a thorough scrubbing, the child feels that something awful has taken place. He does not have the intellectual ability to piece together all the separate factors in the total experience, and to identify what goes on. He only knows that there is something very wrong about feces and that mother's approval is not gained by paying any more attention to it.

The child who has well begun the task of differentiating himself and his mother, and who is carrying over the process of differentiating aspects of other whole experiences that come to his attention, cannot proceed to the current task in learning when anxiety is great and requires exclusive focusing upon what brings approval. He is confused and does not know what has taken place but his power to explore, being disapproved, is no longer available to him. He must again count on his mother to decide for him in a situation in which eventually he could decide for himself. The mother's behavior is an interference to his wishes to explore and to identify his own product, and the child will react to it as to any other frustration. Or, the child may experience opposing goals, such as the wish to express his power further and the need to feel safe and dependent upon his mother. The child may vacillate from one to the other and, being unable to decide, may block in his growth and develop compliant or openly rebellious behavior.

Every child will learn to accept interference as inevitable, reasonable, perhaps useful life experience if personality is not threatened and if anxiety and conflict are not generated through the use of mother love as a barter in the learning process. Yet, it is this bartering element that is sometimes observable in mother and child relations. "If you will go to the bathroom for me, I will like you more or I will give you a lollipop" is often the kind of bribe that is used to bring about compliant behavior. At the time the child is showing heightened interest in bowel function and his new ability to express power in producing through his own body, normally, hostility toward a parent is also felt. The parent who cannot accept that hostility, as a normal element of the child's increasing differentiation of self, and who needs to extinguish its expression immediately, interferes with the child's way of relating to her in his own right.

Centering interferences around the ability to express power, in bowel action as well as in verbal behavior, is a way of forcing the child to feel that he is powerless. Unconditional mother love, respect for the child's emergent biological ability as a newly acquired and important step in the direction of eventual self-control, faith that the child will pattern its behavior along that of the parent where there is a useful relationship between them, and absence of approval or disapproval—these are the principles that permit the child to focus on the learning and to organize along ever more productive lines. When the parent approves the child's interest or when she disapproves it, she stops the child from going forward. A nonjudgmental attitude, such as, "I see, you had a bowel movement," aids the child to identify what the experience is without attaching any special significance to it.

As the child notes that his parents go into the bathroom, and perhaps explores with them the purpose of their trip, he takes on their ways of attending to his bowel functions. The child, however, is likely to have accidents or failures, even when he is trying to use his power to become more like his mother in his toilet activities. Indicating to the child real appreciation for his failures is essential since recognition of failure and the differentiation of failure and success is beginning to dawn in the awareness of the child. A mother can say, "You meant to go to the bathroom but it came too soon; I will clean it up." Or, "You wanted to do it right but you had an accident," is another way of letting the child know that you appreciate his intentions and appreciate the difficulties without showing approval or disapproval.

Delaying satisfaction of wants, connected with bowel functions, is learned when there is a warm relationship between mother and child in which the child is free to communicate what he honestly feels. The child can be himself. He can use his powers to improve himself at his own rate of speed as he takes in his mother's attitudes. Interferences to wants and wishes can also be learned by permitting the child to participate in making decisions that require changes in ongoing activities. Thus, in the morning, a mother can review with the child what will take place. Johnny will have breakfast and then he will play while Mother works around the house, then both will go to the store, then lunch and afterward a nap. After the nap Johnny will have a piece of candy. Asking the child to delay having a piece of candy until after taking a nap is not made so that the child will learn permanently that candy follows an afternoon siesta but that the concept of delay or interference to wants can be gradually learned as plans are made before the want appears. The child learns in small ways to defer his wishes to those of others and at the same time he does not adopt wholly conforming behavior. He learns to structure his life in terms of periods when play and all of his wishes can be granted and other periods when the wishes of others take precedence. Preplanning a day's activities with a child makes it possible for him to express his differentiation from his mother in that he contributes his wishes. The child's behavior gradually comes to include interferences and limits he helps to formulate and subsequently places upon his own behavior.

A child can use his newly acquired power to enhance relations with his mother, or it can be used to disunite them.

Relations are improved when the child's ability is respected and permitted to operate in its natural setting. Relations between mother and child become strained when the child gives up his power and develops compliance, in response to excessive insistence on a schedule for having a bowel movement and when the product is treated with shame and disgust. Relations are also strained when the child resists the mother's commands and retains the stool as a way of showing his rebellion. He can keep his mother waiting a long time and thus control the situation by using his anal power to defeat her. At the same time he can retain his own pleasure as long as he retains the stool and does not comply with commands that his mother cannot enforce. The important point is not that the child must learn to become toilet trained as his mother wishes, but that their relations are distorted and that he must gear all of his activities in the direction of feeling safe with her, rather than in feeling satisfaction in the accomplishment of what he is able to do on his own.

During the second year of life the meaning of events to the child begins to develop rather rapidly. There is already a backlog of felt-relations that help to define the meaning of events to him, but the child does not yet have the vocabulary or the experiences required to interpret events as adults do. He interprets everything that happens to him in terms of what he feels about it. This is a period of *autistic invention, during which all events have a highly personal meaning to him.* These meanings can only be corroborated in talking over what has transpired with others, but the child is very limited in his ability to make clear what his feelings are and how he perceives events. Nevertheless, he "knows" what he feels and his feelings serve as the only guide to the meaning of events; regardless of what adults tell him to think he retains his own private meanings of what happens. The child will communicate the feelings that he has if he feels free to do so, and if he perceives that his expressions will be accorded proper respect. If they are laughed away and he is chided for entertaining thoughts that have not occurred to adults around him he may find it necessary to continue to interpret events on his own, without validating them with others.

The highly personal meaning of the product of bowel action is most often revealed in data provided by psycho-analysts; it is also available to any nurse who works with psychiatric patients who will take the time to note the autistic inventions of patients and to desymbolize them for their underlying meanings. The patient cannot be forthright about expressing the meaning of events and so often uses a highly disguised way of saying what is felt. Nurses can speculate on the meaning and often come close to what it actually means to the patient.

To the young child undergoing toilet training, who cannot understand his mother's failure to appreciate his newly identified power, feces may come to be looked upon as dangerous substances. He does not know why he was whisked away to the bathtub or why the toilet was flushed when he was examining the product, but the look on his mother's face and the way she acted communicated that he was approaching something very dangerous from which she would save him. His mother's pleasure and overwhelming approval when the child is able to produce a bowel movement at the suggested moment leads to other meanings for the child. He begins to feel that there is something magic about having a bowel movement and that he can control his mother's approval in this way—by being good.[2] On the other hand, there is something bad about the magic of bowel movements but he is not clear what that is about.

Learning to acquire ordinary cleanliness is a complex process. Premature training and excessive demands on the child are felt as frustrating experiences and often lead to a clash between the newly acquired power of the child and the mother's power over him. During the entire experience the

[2] See also: Spock and Huschka, *op. cit.* H. S. Sullivan, *The Meaning of Anxiety in Psychiatry and in Life* (Washington, D.C., William Alanson White Psychiatric Foundation), pamphlet, pp. 11-12.

child has only three courses of action open to him: (1) He can be permitted to adapt his needs to those of the family group and gradually learn to deposit his stool where parents with whom he identifies go for the same purpose. (2) He can give up feelings of power and comply with commands, permitting his mother full control of his bodily functions according to her will. (3) He can refuse to give up his power and use it to retain the stool, to withhold his product from others, and thus to defeat their efforts to make him feel powerless. In the latter two courses of action interpersonal relations are distorted and the personality of the child is formed accordingly.[3]

Learning to delay satisfaction in nursing

Both the first and the second psychological tasks discussed constitute focal points in psychobiological development around which each child learns something about the nature of his relatedness to others. What is learned is often carried over into later life. In situations where patients find it difficult to accept the reality of illness, as interference to the normal course of life activities, they often find it difficult to defer wants and wishes that seemingly lessen the promotion of experiences leading to health. Such patients present seriously challenging problems in nursing. Whether the interference is perceived as a frustration leading to open aggression toward the nurse or members of the health team or to covert aggression in the form of idling hostility, apathy, or self-destructive trends, these patients all tax the ingenuity, understanding, and patience of nurses. Patients who have not developed ability to accept interference in any form or to delay gratification of wants and wishes, which are often poorly visualized, are rarely able to show appreciation for

[3] See also: Max Levin, "Delay (Pavlov) in Human Physiology," *The American Journal of Psychiatry*, Vol. 102, No. 4 (January, 1946), p. 483. A discussion of physiological aspects of delay. Mabel Huschka, "The child's response to coercive bowel training," *Psychosomatic Medicine*, 4:301-308 (1942).

kindness shown should the nurse entertain this expectation from them. Nurses who resent "being taken for granted" find it difficult to sustain a helping relation in these events.

When assisting the patient in making use of illness as an experience in which learning and further personality development can take place, nurses must be able to understand and to cope with their own feelings regarding "difficult patients" in order to develop experiences that develop fruitful interpersonal relations. The nurse who adheres to a rigid plan of operation and has difficulty in permitting patients to intrude their goals into her plans must come to recognize these as interferences to her own wants and needs, to her own inability to defer in a professional way to the wants of patients. Patients are less powerful particularly in the hospital situation and it is sometimes difficult to acknowledge interferences from less powerful individuals than the nurse.

It is helpful to have a picture of the structure of character encountered in patients who have failed in completing the second psychological task successfully.[4] This assists the nurse in differentiating those patients who transitorily are disturbed by an unexpected interfering event and those whose character demands certain kinds of behavior. Fromm has suggested types and clues to the kind of behavior likely to be manifested.[5] (1) There are individuals who are exploitative, manipulating others in order to achieve their own ends, while at the same time they are unable to be productive in their own right. Others are held suspect, are looked upon with envy and jealousy, and are used to vent hostility in a way that enhances the exploiter. (2) There are individuals who feel safe only when they can hoard, withhold from others, and count their possessions as their own. While they are orderly to a fault and punctual about appointments, for example, they find it impossible to share their feelings or ideas or their

---

[4] For full discussion see: Patrick Mullahy, *Oedipus: Myth and Complex* (New York, Hermitage House, Inc., 1948), pp. 261-62. Also: Erich Fromm, *Man for Himself* (New York, Farrar and Rinehart, Inc., 1949).

[5] See chart p. 217.

goods with others; thus they are unable to relate to others for it would mean giving of themselves. (3) A third type is referred to by Fromm as the marketer, who can vary outward relations with people in terms of what has selling value. The variations are so great that they seem to be without a structure in personality that is stable and relatively consistent.

Horney describes similar character traits, laying stress on individuals who strive constantly to exert control over others and to be right, becoming seriously discomforted when errors in judgment are made. A second type pointed out is the individual who retains and seeks to hide his possessions, being unable to share private experiences with others.[6]

The problem arises as to how the professional nurse can relate to patients whose behavior implies the character traits underlying it, as indicated above. A great deal depends upon the amount of insight the nurse has into her own character traits, and to the way she relates to others—the motivations that operate below the conventional reasons that she gives for choosing to be a nurse. White suggests that it is most difficult to modify the behavior of human beings, who cannot modify their own, except in a treatment situation. However, he concludes that when we act "as if" difficulties were not insurmountable, and "as if" they could be modified, that it is remarkable what changes can be observed to take place.[7]

There are no hard and fast rules to be followed. A nurse who has a productive orientation to life will use her ingenuity to find ways to help patients to feel safe enough so that they can become aware of and thus examine their relations with her. A number of experiences documented by nurses illustrate what is possible.

Mrs. Smith is an adult arthritic patient who has a very strong wish to dominate situations and people. Every time nurses are changed it takes her several weeks to get used to

[6] Karen Horney, *New Ways in Psychoanalysis* (New York, W. W. Norton & Company, 1939), p. 74.

[7] William A. White, *Twentieth Century Psychiatry* (New York, W. W. Norton & Company, Inc., 1936), p. 137.

the new nurse. She always demands complete care which includes bath, shampoo, and haircut, whenever she decides these are necessary. She wants her nails trimmed properly and her bunion pads applied at just the right angle. She prefers her bath in the morning, preferably between ten-thirty and eleven-thirty.

The nurse tries to meet her demands whenever possible. On occasion emergencies arise and it is not possible to meet all of her demands. They have found that she is more amenable to having her nursing care given at any hour of the day than in eliminating any step of it. Thus, they try to accede to one or two of her needs and satisfy these completely and find that she is then more willing to delay some of her demands until the emergency is over. They have found that talking it over with her when the emergency arises, and planning with her when her needs can be met, is a better way than letting all of her needs go unmet. Also, as the patient expresses cues that indicate that she is ready to take on any small part of her daily activities the nurse responds to these in a nonjudgmental way; that is, she neither approves or disapproves but merely remarks, "You want to do it yourself, very well."

It is noteworthy that the patient was able to accept interferences to her wishes when she participated in the revision of plans for her.

Mrs. Brown was an attractive thirty-eight-year-old mother who spoke only Greek. She was hospitalized for suspected lymphosarcoma of the left ankle. Her family managed to get her to come to the hospital by telling her that she would only have to stay for a few days. As the days stretched into weeks she became restless, was frequently found crying, and eagerly awaited visits from her family. She expressed many reasons why she should go home. Finally an operation was performed and the diagnosis was confirmed, which meant a longer hospital stay than had been predicted and further operations. The patient assumed that the worst was over after the operation and when she was faced with the reality of her

problem she became argumentative, sullen, tearful, and refused to accept the new goal. She insisted that she was going
home. Finally a two-week visit was arranged.

After two weeks the patient was readmitted for the complete operation and subsequent nursing. She was more con-
tented, participated in taking care of herself, was generous
with other patients, and in general accepted the reality of
her medical problem.

[In this experience we can see how unreal goals are set
when families mean to be kind to a member. All subsequent
goals that need to be set in order to meet the needs of the
problem act as interferences to the patient's goal and are
reacted to with hostility and aggression, direct and indirect.
When the patient was permitted the satisfaction of her goal—
going home—she could take in more recent evidence and
vary her goal accordingly. Once the goal of full recovery was
accepted by her, she could harness her activities to co-operation in meeting her own goal with help. The trip home reduced her feelings of powerlessness and the satisfaction it
afforded relieved her anxiety to a point where she could
vary her goal in the light of experience.]

A third experience has to do with a three-and-one-half-year-
old child, whose personality is undergoing formation. He
was admitted to the hospital and operated for correction of
webbed fingers of both hands. Following surgery, the child
continued to suck his finger and thumb, as he had been accustomed to doing before surgery. In order to discourage this
practice the nurse bandaged his hands rather heavily. However, the child's need to suck was so strong that he managed
to get through the bandages and contaminate the operative
areas. Restraints were then used, the child protesting vigor-
ously by screaming and kicking. The nurse left the room
and when she returned she found the child smearing feces
over himself, from head to toe, at the same time eating the
fecal material. Again the dressings were contaminated and
required changing. Finally the physician put plaster casts on
the child at each elbow, after which the child expressed first

rage and later complete apathy. This response was short lived for the child soon found a way to get to his hands and to express his need to suck.

All of the nursing care was oriented toward preventing the child from contaminating the area. The behavior of the child, as an expression of a very strong need to suck, was not understood and consequently substitutive sucking possibilities were not offered. There is no evidence to show how completely the child felt the separation from his mother, or the extent to which his need to suckle had been thwarted as an infant. But here was an instance where nurses might have produced a nursing bottle, a lollipop, pretzels, zwieback, a pacifier, toys, or many other possibilities for the child to both gratify his need to suck and harness the energy derived from tension into some other activities. Each nursing measure was a new interference that intensified his feelings of frustration. The strength of the drive may be inferred from its persistent expression. At one point the child moved forward to another area of pleasure, smearing, and this too was thwarted in a rather traumatic way. The child had no alternative except to struggle to gratify his needs on his own or to give up his needs and a satisfaction response. The evidence does not show how much time was spent by nurses in helping him to develop a feeling of belonging in the new situation, but it is evident that he was thrown back upon himself for the satisfaction of his needs, that he could not count on others for help in this situation—only for interferences to his wishes.

Another experience shows how the goals of the treatment plan are looked upon as an interference to achievement of satisfaction, when a warm relationship between nurse and patient has not been developed before treatment activities are outlined for the patient. A ten-year-old boy with diabetes was admitted to the hospital. He had been diabetic since the age of six and developed a nephritis, which necessitated hospitalization. During the acute stage of illness there was no difficulty in controlling the sugar level and insulin requirements but during convalescence the sugar present in urine and blood was uncontrollable. The diet was checked, frequent urinalysis was done, a quantitative urinalysis was made, the other children in the ward were questioned as to the boy's activities, but nothing could be found that would account for the new development. Finally, one of the other patients admitted that he was going to give the diabetic patient some candy for beating up another kid when the nurses weren't looking. Then the nurses became conscious of the fact that the diabetic patient had been distant with nurses, rarely confiding in them, and often after a treatment was performed he would fail to respond to questions for long periods of time. Once the nurses realized that they did not have a useful relationship with the patient and that he actually resented them, they made an effort to come to know him as a person. As the child began to feel accepted despite his difficulties the nurses began to communicate to him what was involved in his medical problem and together they worked out ways for meeting the demands of the problem. Being accepted by nurses, the patient was able to give up his practice of intimidating the other boys in the ward and began to take a real interest in becoming a member of the group. He taught his mother what was necessary for his care when he got home.

In this experience the nurses had not helped the patient to move from a completely dependent relationship to one in which he could accept interferences to his wishes. It is not enough to offer unconditional care. As the patient shows cues to growth, interest in what is happening to him and what is required of him, the nurse can respond in ways that make it possible for the patient to move forward. This movement always necessitates examination of the patient's feelings about his present difficulty. The nurses in this instance were most likely overprotective while the patient was ill and then took it for granted that he had learned all that was necessary and that he would comply with plans outlined for him. The child felt the overprotectiveness as a smothering kind of relationship and once he gained freedom from it expressed his hostility, felt with interferences to his growth, by defeating the goals of the professional team. As the patient became aware of what was happening to him, and as nurses made it possible for him to express his feelings about treatments, he could get clearer on the meaning of events and release his ability to co-operate.

When a professional nurse has managed to assist a patient with needs for dependence and to lessen the strength of a longing for dependency, the patient reaches a phase in the relationship where interference or delay must intervene to some of the patient's wishes. This is often necessary from the standpoint of administrative policy—since there are new and sicker patients being admitted every day. More important, it is necessary as a factor in helping the patient to become more self-directing in relation to his problems. The patient must be able to share what is available in the form of services —nursing time and materials.

Sharing is a component part of the ability to accept interference from others and to delay needs and wants in consideration of the interests and needs of others. It is a difficult social concept that is not learned in childhood in most instances, as a result of its being taught prematurely as a dogmatic assertion to be accepted: "You must share with others." Particularly, when acceptance of the sharing concept is coerced by threats to personality, such as, "Other children won't play with you if you don't share your toys," is the adapted acceptance likely to be traumatic. Reinforcement of the need to resist consideration of the needs of others and to protect the interests of the self are ways of feeling safe when personality is threatened.

Sharing is a natural expression of willingness to divide or give up possessions actually owned. It operates only under conditions of freedom from coercion and is not synonymous with coerced giving up of things according to standards that seem to operate for others. Steps in the choice process in the sharing concept include: (1) Inner security that is sufficient for asserting, "It's mine," and for protecting that property against confiscation. (2) Evolution of ability to say, "I'm using it, I'll be through with it shortly, and then you may have it. (3) Eventual ability to say, "Let's talk it over," to express and discuss differences and reach consensuses or plans; to consider who "owns" it, who had it first, who needs it most, and the reasons for wanting it now. (4) Ability to recognize needs of others anticipatorily and to volunteer one's own property or abilities for use by other more needful individuals.

Hoarding of food, soap, toilet paper is often a "major issue" in nursing patients in large general and psychiatric hospital wards where dispossessed patients cling to these small "things" as semblances of ownership. There are individuals who recognize *who they are* by what they have, or own, and for many ward patients this may be evidenced in hoarding scraps of bread. It would be well worth the effort required of nurses in these situations to assist the patient to protect his hoard, in the case of food, by providing plastic bags or cans so that vermin won't despoil the hoard. An interesting and useful experiment in human behavior could develop from large-scale study of this problem in a ward situation. The value of the hoard increases to the degree that it is not permitted openly, aided, and abetted by the nursing staff as an expression of character to reinforce feelings of security in the patient. Only when the patient learns, for sure, that he can feel safe despite his hoard will he give up the practice of storing up a crust of bread for some future impoverishment of personality.

Unconditional interest and acceptance on the part of the nurse is an essential part of observation which leads the nurse to a basis for understanding the patient and for fostering his growth. When the nurse and patient have developed rapport, that is, largely understand each other's preconceptions and expectations, it is possible for the nurse anticipatorily to suggest interferences and delays in meeting needs and requests. Where there is a relationship of acceptance plans may be formulated together that will be in the interest of the patient's growth and the solution of his problem.

Summary

Interferences to wishes are inevitable in life and during an illness in which nursing is counted upon for valuable help. Nurses can aid patients to accept interference when they are cognizant of it and of the character traits that operate to distort interpersonal relations. When nurses are able to demonstrate and thus communicate acceptance of the patient as he is, and when there is an understanding between them of each other's preconceptions about people and expectations about health services, the nurse is able to formulate plans with the patient that include his goals with regard to the problem. When nurses are unable to recognize that patients sometimes interfere with the nurse's wants and wishes, they cannot help patients relying on professional assistance to delay satisfaction. As in early childhood training, nurses can get conforming behavior or rebellious outbursts when the needs and feelings of the patient are not permitted full expression and taken into account in what is done in the situation. Unless the patient is permitted to use his powers, in his own way, at his own rate of speed, he is powerless. Nurses who aid patients to feel safe and secure, so that wants can be expressed and satisfaction eventually achieved, also help them to strengthen personal power that is needed for productive social activities.

CHAPTER 10

Identifying Oneself

Overview

EVERYONE HAS a mental picture of himself that operates when he relates to other individuals. This view of self is not inherited but develops in the social milieu in which biological constitution and capacities are expressed and rewarded or punished by adults in the situation. When an individual learns to count on others for help when it is needed and to accept delays in the satisfaction of wishes and desires, a view of self that includes getting and giving operates in relations with others. A third psychological task that all children face is that of becoming more aware of their identity, getting clearer on responses to the question: Who am I? The purpose of this chapter is to provide background information on how children grapple with this task and to show views of self that emerge. Every patient has a concept of self that operates to improve or to distort interpersonal relations with professional persons. Every nurse has a view of self that is expressed in her relations with patients in ways that facilitate or hinder the growth of both parties in the situation. In this chapter operations of the self-concept will be shown in relation to problems that arise when the third psychological task is not completed or when it is reactivated in situations in which an individual is ill.

Essential questions

How does a child come to identify who he is? How does he learn to differentiate who he is and who others in the situation are? What difference does it make if he is able to identify himself or not? Does it make a person more egotistical and self-centered to know who he is and what he is capable of doing? How does the evolution of the concept of self occur when there are obstacles that seem overwhelming, such as physiological dysfunctioning at birth and gross psychological rejection during early years of personality formation? Is the young child able to evolve a concept of self without receiving genuine respect as a person from other adults in the social milieu? What can be done to help a patient, confined to a hospital for long-term illness, to expand a meager concept of self? Is there a role to be taken by nurses that will aid patients to recognize and to change their view of themselves? Should nurses consider a new way of viewing what are thought to be the more mechanical functions of nursing, namely, washing, feeding, and giving treatments to patients as prescribed? More recently, great emphasis has been placed upon the nurse giving total care to the patient; to what extent is this possible? What is involved and how can a nurse care for the patient as a whole? These vital questions provide a framework for discussion that will lead nurses to clarify their thinking in a way that permits and aids them to determine roles that they can take in relations with patients.

Personality formation in childhood: background information

In order to understand the interaction that takes place when the concept of self that operates for a nurse and for her patient enters into their relationship in the sickroom, it is necessary to look back upon the way personality is formed in early childhood. The need for receiving unconditional mother love, as a step in learning to count on others for help, has already been discussed (Chapter 8). The need for experiencing the respect of others as the child discovers and begins to exercise new powers in relation to biological functioning, in a way that aids him to learn to delay his wish for satisfaction as he learns to take into account social conventions and the wishes of others, has also been discussed (Chapter 9). These two tasks comprise a partial differentiation of the world and the child's view of himself in it. There is necessity to spread the foundation for adult productive functioning across a broader base by completing further the differentiation of self as separated from but related to others.

A concept of self develops as a product of interaction with adults. At first the child refers to himself as "Johnnie does it" or "Me do it." These are first steps to a more mature expression as in "I can do that." Through the ways that others take care of the child, anticipatory reactions or expectations of others are set up. The child learns to expect that his communication of discomfort or a need, through crying or verbal behavior, will lead to feelings of satisfaction as a mother or her surrogate responds to his cues for help. He may find that his communications will be ignored, that satisfaction will not be forthcoming; a new need, to feel safe, arises, and the child will discover that he feels safer and less anxious when he does not ask for anything from his mother. In either instance a concept of self begins to form. When the child's cues are heeded he can begin to think in terms of, "I am a person who can say what is needed and get satisfaction through the help of others who respect me." When the child's relations with his mother require him to be unconditional, to make no demands upon her, a very different set of expectations are learned. The view of self is more likely to be in the direction of, "Others will take care of me if I remain helpless and do not ask for anything." The more active child may rebel against conditional relations with his mother, using his powers to defeat her at the same time he is enhancing his own feelings of power. The view of self that develops is in the direction of, "I'll get mine first without help from anyone."

The three variations in viewing oneself may be summarized: (1) "I can identify my wants and needs, communicate them to others who respect me, and get assistance as it is needed to achieve satisfaction." (2) "I do not need to identify my wants; if I remain helpless others will give me what they think I need and I will feel safe then; a helpless person who makes no demands cannot be deserted." (3) "I cannot count on others to give me any kind of assistance; they do not respect me or my abilities, but I will get what I need without help; I will take it if necessary."

These views of self arise out of relations with adults in the family situation and are more or less reinforced in relations with other adults in the neighborhood, in schools, in other social institutions. *Primary skills in living are learned, in relation to taking food, elimination of wastes, cleanliness, and avoidance of dangerous situations. At the same time, the child observes how others feel about him as a person and begins to structure the roles he will take in relation to them and to the world as he views it.* When the expectations of others are perceived to include more or less permanent roles as infant or child, being helpless in deciding against parental or adult domination that at the same time ensures feelings of safety, the child has less opportunity to vary his roles in accordance with changing chronological and psychological ages and the behavior that society expects. When the expectations of others are perceived to include roles that are more mature than what is possible, biologically and psychologically, at various age levels the child ensures feelings of safety by adapting too fast, and thus is denied the opportunity to savor satisfaction of emotional and growth needs at each level. The child views himself as an adult, when adult control of his feelings is demanded of him before he has experienced the feeling of being a child.

Sullivan holds that the self becomes "circumscribed by reflected appraisals," as processes of maturation and learning proceed from infancy through childhood to adulthood.[1] The child takes cues from adults in the situation who are significant to him.[2] As he is permitted to do so, the child will respond to his own cues using behavior that is appropriate to his feelings; when adults can permit the child freedom in improving upon his responses at his own rate of speed and as a result of experiences with children of his own age, the child learns skills for reorganization of his behavior and reconstruction of his experience. When the child is not permitted this freedom, and the adult is guided by the assumption that the child must be told what to think and how to act, the child acquires skills in being compliant to the demands of others. *The ways in which adults appraise the child and the way he functions in relation to his experiences and perceptions are taken in or introjected and become the child's view of himself.*

During the genital phase of psychosexual development the cultural views on sexual activities, their meaning and consequences in life often enter into the attitudes an adult expresses toward the growing child. The child has not yet undergone the many experiences that would aid in illuminating discoveries in relation to pleasant stimulation afforded in manipulation of the genitals, and therefore cannot appreciate what an adult might feel about genital play. The child only knows that he has just discovered a heretofore unnoticed part of himself, his *genitalia,* and that pleasurable feelings occur when his hands stimulate this part of his body.

The genital region is equipped with tissue that is highly sensitive and that affords pleasant sensations when touched, in much the same fashion as the mucous membranes of the mouth and lips and the anus can be stimulated in a pleasurable way. When the child first discovers these satisfactions afforded by his own body, he will *explore* them further as a way of differentiating all that makes up parts of himself and

[1] Patrick Mullahy, *Oedipus: Myth and Complex* (New York, Hermitage House, Inc., 1948), p. 297.
[2] See also Fig. 3, p. 21.

his body through which the self expresses its functions. If the child is deprived of meeting other needs, for affection, for feeling close to his mother, for exploring, manipulating, and using his toys in his own way, the child will *exploit* these bodily areas as outlets for feelings of comfort not afforded in any other way.

Every child will indulge in genital play at some time, just as every child will test objects that are new and interesting by putting them in his mouth or will smear feces in order to become fully acquainted with the product of his own body. Permitting the child to make these discoveries and to explore them to the extent needed for clarity of what is involved and at the same time making available in the situation other new and exciting media that can be explored and manipulated is a way of making it possible for the child to transfer the heightened sense of usefulness that accompanies discovery of genitals onto objects that are also satisfying for the child's curiosity.

Many mothers and mother surrogates have preconceptions about sex play in children that operate and compel them to deny the child the opportunity for rounding out his "body image" as an aspect of the concept of self that he is gaining. Many adults focus their attention on disapproving the child's natural interest in his body and consequently cannot focus on other possibilities that could be made available to the child, such as toys, lumps of clay, finger paints, poster paints, etc. In the past, masturbation has been thought of as a threat to "sanity" and a practice to be curbed at once, at all costs. *A child who is not provided with opportunities for transferring his creative interests from his body to other objects in the situation, in a climate that leaves him free to do so,* is likely to find ways to masturbate in secret and thus gain personal feelings of pleasure that he is denied in his relations with people.

A climate in which a child is free to decide which outlet provides greater satisfaction is one in which materials are made available and the child is not coerced into or hampered in using them in his own way. There is a difference between diverting the child's attention from sexual activities and developing the situation in such a way that he will gradually wish to divert himself. The harm in masturbation is not in the act itself but in the feelings of guilt that are generated in the child when he is forced to deny the discovery of sexual parts. All children will want to experience genital excitation, to find out what is involved in it for them, and will want to go on to make use of the heightened sense of usefulness that arises with discovery of genitals. That is, they will put aside their interest in body parts willingly as other new experiences in which they can explore their abilities further are made available for them.

When the preconceptions of a parent or surrogate operate to deny the child the opportunity to choose his course of action, the sexual drive is overstimulated or repressed or dissociated from awareness. Its usefulness to the individual, for later creative activities on a biological or symbolical level, may be permanently unavailable unless psychotherapeutic intervention occurs. The genital area, genital functions, and the larger meaning of creativity in a symbolic way give rise to anxiety and thus may become functions to be avoided; the view of self that the child holds cannot include these functions when they are dissociated from the self that operates in awareness. However, the sexual drive continues to work outside of awareness and modes of living include acts that take place without conscious control of the individual. Sexual perversions, delinquency, all are ways of acting out sexual and other drives and needs that function in dissociation.

When a child discovers genital body parts his goal is to find out to his satisfaction what is involved. Adult preconceptions and attempts to coerce the child into doing something else are felt as interferences to this goal; the child feels frustrated and will respond in one of the three ways that

Zones of interaction and needs involved	Pattern of mothering experiences—some examples	Acquired needs	Concept of self that emerges	Acquired motivating forces in the self
ORAL: Feeding	Permits "self-demand." Provides unconditional mother love.	"Positive groping." Wish to struggle in relative comfort. Wish to seek help when needed.	I am what I can get through my own efforts for others will help me.	Wish to struggle to express wants and needs. Seeking and use of help when needed.
ANAL: Bowel action	Permits self-training when ready. Avoids harsh interferences with wishes. Is sensitive to self-expressions and permits even hostile ones.	To permit the body to act for itself.	I am what I can do, produce, through my own efforts. Sustained bodily integrity.	Wish to do, to give to others, to produce, to contribute.
GENITAL: Sex interest and curiosity, as aspects of self-discovery	Permits early exploration of body parts. Provides varied media in situation to which child can turn when ready. Answers questions related to sex discovery. Permits positive feelings about sex.	To know body and parts of self. To reproduce and to create. To feel safe while inquiring freely. To differentiate self further in basis of new discoveries about self and world.	I am what I do, feel, produce, think, create. I am free to act, to make choices, to love others. I have wants and I can identify and satisfy them. I am related to others who respect me as a person.	Wish for self-expression. Ability to doubt, inquire, take risks, to find out, to sustain, delay in satisfactions, to go on to new experiences in comfort, willingly.

Fig. 9. Mothering experiences that have positive weight in total personality formation and functioning.

Zones of interaction and needs involved	Pattern of mothering experiences—some examples	Acquired needs	Concept of self that emerges	Acquired motivating forces in the self
ORAL: Feeding	Clock feeding. Cries ignored. Fear of "spoiling" the infant.	To struggle in vain. Refusal to struggle; apathy. To overemphasize struggle. Passive receptivity.	I am what others are willing to give me for not struggling. I have to struggle alone; I can't trust others to help.	Wish to be taken care of; to be helpless in order to get attention. Wish to get more, get it first.
ANAL: Bowel action	Trained when adults decide and methods adults insist upon. Adult wishes interfere with child wishes.	To compel the body to act in compliance with demands. To force action—compulsive use of cathartics. To submit to or rebel against authority and power of others.	I am what I have, own, possess, can barter with. Others respect me for my possessions. I am what I can make myself do as others command it.	Wish to comply, to withhold, to hoard, to exploit.
GENITAL: Self-interest and curiosity as an aspect of self-discovery	Repressive and guilt provoking commands to the child. Feelings of shame aroused in the child. Threats and fear used to control sex play.	To hide and avoid knowing all parts of self. To feel secure in "not doing." To manage anxiety by avoiding self and feelings.	I am "good" because I avoid what others forbid. Uncritical acceptance of values of others. Isolation from others on the basis of unworthiness.	Wish for self-negation. Doubting leads to anxiety. Avoidance of all risks.

Fig. 10.   Mothering experiences that have negative weight in total personality formation and functioning.

217

individuals respond to frustration.[3] When the child has already experienced many forms of punishment or threats in this direction, two goals may be set up: to explore the new discovery and to achieve satisfaction or to feel safe with a parent who has heretofore threatened or meted out punishment. A conflict occurs. Depending upon the degree of anxiety that arises, as the child begins to contemplate what the parent (who may or may not be present) will do, and upon the previous pattern of responding when discomfort is felt, the child may follow a number of courses of action. He may block in his activities; he may vacillate between what he expects his mother wants and what he wishes to do; he may use ways that worked earlier in getting satisfactions, such as smearing feces or thumb sucking. In his relations with his mother, and with other children, he may strengthen his feelings of helplessness, moving toward his mother for greater protection and care at the same time he is giving up his own wishes to struggle and explore his world. Or, he may move further away from people, becoming more withdrawn and isolated from them, often by intensifying his interest in one aspect of play that can be accomplished alone. When frustration, conflict, and/or anxiety enter into the child's experiences before he has useful skills for overcoming obstacles and making choices full evolution of capacities cannot take place.

The child takes in the attitudes of others around him by way of his feelings. He empathizes what others feel concerning him. He takes cues from their gestures, their acts toward him, their facial expressions. The child is always more powerless than the adults and thus needs to rely upon them for clues that ensure him that he is accepted and respected. The child lacks the strength and the skills that are required for evaluating the validity and correctness of attitudes that others manifest toward him. Consequently, appraisals that adults make enter into the view of self that a child develops in more or less uncritical fashion. Experiences that occur later

[3] See p. 95.

in life may aid in the modification of a view of self that is held, or, they may reinforce a negative view and thus impede further progress.[4]

In Sullivan's theory of interpersonal relations the "self-dynamism" has three aspects: (1) the self that is readily available in awareness; (2) selectively inattended components that are available to recall; (3) dissociated elements of self that are excluded more or less permanently from awareness but operate in covert fashion.[5] The self-system is thus conceived as an operating motivational system on three levels, some aspects of which operate consciously in interpersonal relations while others operate marginally or without conscious control of the individual. These concepts of Sullivan's are roughly comparable to those of Freud, namely, preconscious, conscious, and unconscious, but they cannot be considered as identical. There seems to be an operational difference in that Sullivan's conceptualization lends itself more readily to visualizing what is actually happening in an interpersonal relationship.[6]

The concept of self is related to ongoing learning of all three psychological tasks but overconcern about the sexual drive often distorts relations between mother and child to an extent that the child feels "cut off" from communications with others. When a child needs to focus all of his activities in the direction of getting and sustaining approval, or avoiding anxiety connected with disapproval, from parents and surrogates, his concept of self cannot expand beyond what works and is acceptable to the adults upon whom he must count for feelings of safety or security. Thus if a little girl discovers that the genitals of a little boy are different from her own, but cannot communicate this to her mother and review her feelings about it, her perception of being "cut off" in her relations with her mother is expanded in her

[4] H. S. Sullivan, *op. cit.*, pp. 297-300.

[5] *Ibid.*

[6] See diagrams presented in: H. S. Sullivan, *The Meaning of Anxiety in Psychiatry and in Life* (Washington, D.C., William Alanson White Psychiatric Foundation), pamphlet, 1948, pp. 6-10.

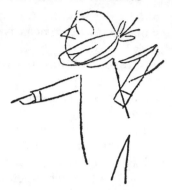

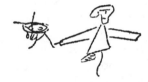

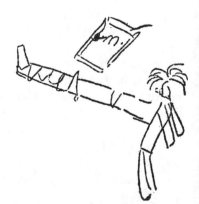

Fig. 11. A fifteen-year-old boy's drawings that show a series of experiences in which he felt "cut off" in various ways.

autistic thinking. It is debatable whether a "castration complex," as described in psychoanalytic literature, will become a devastating perception to a child who can communicate freely what is felt about likes and differences among people as they are observed in everyday experiences. The way in which the feeling of being "cut off" from the tender respect and attention from parents becomes stereotyped and the meaning extended to many other activities in life is illustrated in the drawings of a fifteen-year-old boy who entered a psychiatric hospital with a diagnosis of Schizophrenia, Catatonic type. It can be noticed that he felt "cut off" from communication with others, he felt genital castration when sexual drives were not permitted expression in any form, and a leg infection led to a discussion in which he heard doctors and nurses talking about cutting off his leg. (See Fig. 11, p. 220.)

When an individual feels that he cannot satisfy his curiosity and communicate to others what is experienced he cannot differentiate himself from parental ties, since his need for dependence is strengthened and often becomes a longing. The concept of self that emerges is meager, passive, unproductive. Strecker has elaborated on the seriousness of this problem as a social issue during World War II.[7] When an individual fails to learn adequately to want to take into account the wishes and needs of others, in his relations with adults, exhortation and discussion of ideals does not help. The world of others is not open to perception until an individual becomes aware of his own feelings about it. The demarcation of self, and recognition of ways in which the self is expressed, can occur only when a child is free for discovering and utilizing his capacities. Approval and disapproval, or total indifference, from parents operate to limit, to provide rigid boundaries within which the child can function and feel safe. When the child must concentrate all of his attention on activities that bring approval, or that avoid disapproval, or that bring disapproval as a way of avoiding

[7] Edward Strecker, *Their Mothers' Sons* (Philadelphia, Lippincott, 1946).

being ignored, he is not free to test out experiences that go beyond parental appraisals and that permit focusing on learning to live with people. When the boundaries are constricted with many disapprovals, the expansion of self is limited even further. Fromm attributes the development of poverty in relatedness to others to the failure to develop feelings of self-affirmation, the ability to love oneself being basic to the ability to consider the wishes of others.[8]

The concept of self as seen in nursing situations

The view an individual has of himself is always risked in an interpersonal relationship; it is often unwittingly protected by various forms of behavior. Patients who demand concrete assistance, such as pills, treatments, enemas, often use these demands to protect themselves from expressing longings for dependency in more direct ways. The meaning of behavior in all nursing situations becomes clearer when the view of self that both nurse and patient hold is understood. *The self always responds selectively to experience and is the organizer and integrator of experience.* Snygg and Combs state this as a principle in human behavior.[9] The way behavior looks to another person sheds little light on its meaning and its improvement; what it means to the patient, in terms of his perception of an event, gives clues as to the way it is purposeful to him.

In order to be helpful to patients it is necessary to develop some understanding of how the patient perceives himself, and how he views the situation confronting him. The responses that the patient makes to the nurse, or to treatments, or to various facets in the situation, are always selective with reference to himself. In relating to a patient, the nurse can examine clues in herself, responses called out in her by

[8] Erich Fromm, *Man for Himself* (New York, Farrar and Rinehart, Inc., 1948).

[9] Donald Snygg and Arthur W. Combs, *Individual Behavior* (New York, Harper & Brothers, 1949), pp. 12-13.

this particular patient, and she can work with him for a degree of clarity on how he perceives himself and the presenting medical problem.

Each recurring problem that crops up in life challenges anew that constellation of feelings that makes up a view of self. Each difficulty that presents itself to a patient who is ill mobilizes his total personality as it functions in relation to the presenting problem. While a patient faces different problems in different ways, there is an underlying pattern of responding that is characteristic of the personality of that individual. Shades or intensities of personality or character are expressed as a patient focuses upon a problem that he faces. *A nurse can relate to the patient as a whole, only to the extent that she is capable of seeing his whole personality focused on his problem.* Likewise, the nurse is seen by the patient through the way in which she faces the emergent problem with him. The patient cannot see the nurse as a person who has a family, who makes philanthropic contributions readily, and who willingly shares her possessions with her roommate; he sees her through the attitudes she manifests toward his difficulty as they are perceived by him as helpful or as affronts to him as a person.

The patient's concept of self is interlocked with his problem—it is his, it is an event that is happening to him, it demands revisions in his feelings about himself in the direction of satisfaction or feelings of safety. In order to understand the dynamics that lead to a formation of a concept of self, it is necessary to look at the child-rearing patterns to which the patient might have been exposed. In observing the way in which a patient relates to a nurse, a nurse who has insight into her own operations can get many more clues than are usually given in case histories about patients. She can speculate with lesser or greater accuracy on the meaning of the patient's behavior depending upon the extent to which she can observe herself in the situation, and the patient's responses as being made to her—as an illusory figure or as a person he has come to know and to respect.

Asking questions about how a person views himself usually brings conventional or expected answers. For example, how would student or graduate nurses respond if they were asked to write a one-page paper filling in the meaning of the following incompleted sentence: I AM A PERSON WHO . . . How would each nurse identify who she is? What words would she choose to convey attitudes, feelings, actions, and values that characterize her relations with others? Would nurses tend to put down what was thought to be the expected answers, rather than what was genuinely felt?

Similarly, how would nurses respond if they were asked to complete the following sentence, with reference to a patient, a parent, a classmate, or an instructor in nursing: SHE IS A PERSON WHO . . . Contemplating these exercises gives some clues to the degree of awareness of self that operates and the readiness to make judgments about others that cannot be made about the self. When a nurse is able to go beyond conventional expectations, such as "I am a person who likes people," and when she can be honest about what she really feels, then there is a chance of reorienting feelings that are often unwittingly demonstrated in relations with others.

The nurse's feelings about food and food taking is worthy of examination. How does she look on herself in relation to the act of feeding? Does she have hard and fast convictions about what "eating well" implies? Do these convictions stem from her own past experiences or is there sufficient scientific evidence to show what "eating well" is for all individuals under all possible circumstances? Should a person who is tense and anxious eat as much as a person who is not? What does anxiety do to the processes of assimilation and absorption of food? Does the nurse know what eating or leaving food means to the patient? What are the possible courses of action that will develop the wish to eat for different patients? Leaving the patient's food so that he can eat it without being watched and staying with the patient, as if detached from the feeding situation, are merely two possible courses of action that might promote the wish to eat in the patient. Does vomiting mean that the patient is rejecting food? Can food taking or food rejection symbolize larger meanings, such as rejecting a person who feeds, or the commands or ideas of that individual? Whatever actions the nurse uses in relation to patients who overeat or who refuse to eat are connected with the nurse's view of herself. When her own preconceptions about feeding serve as interferences to the patient's goals, as symbolized in the way the patient eats or does not eat, the wish to eat in support of bodily integrity cannot be developed. The patient may rebel further, redoubling his refusal to eat; or the patient may comply and eat as he is told to do.

The nurse's views on "habit formation" also enter into her relations with patients. Cleanliness is a value that is often stressed in early childhood and reinforced in the school of nursing. While there is merit in cleanliness, rigidity in this area promotes difficulty for the patient. Unless a nurse examines how she feels about dirt and untidiness, with reference to herself, and becomes aware of the way in which her own views restrict the patient, she may distort relations by emphasizing points that were overstressed in the patient's early childhood. For example, the psychotic patient who has had to become seriously ill in order to free himself to reject interferences, particularly with reference to exploration of smearing feces, may be pushed back still further by emphasis on cleanliness by nurses. The removal of inhibiting disapproval patterns, the escape from commands of disapproving familial figures, may be a first step in personality expansion. When the nurse insists on cleanliness and order and makes demands upon patients that are felt as interferences to newly visualized goals, the interference may reverse the processes of self-repair and self-renewal. This is a difficult concept for nurses to accept since it seems to negate all that is known about asepsis, but, perhaps the antibiotics will provide security and reparative procedures that will permit relaxation of standards of cleanliness when this is necessary for personality reconstruction and the reorganization of a patient's past experience.

It is at this point in nursing that medical method and psychiatric method are essentially different. While a nurse is often called upon to educate a patient about a disease condition and the medical facts on which he can base certain controls that will ameliorate or improve that condition, the same educational procedure does not pertain when the patient's feelings and thoughts are given consideration. Therapeutic procedure in psychiatry is merely a vehicle through which the patient is enabled to clarify and reconstruct feelings, thoughts, and ideals already held. Other social institutions—education, religion, the press, and radio—may openly present and discuss social values and various ways of thinking, feeling, and acting in relation to them. While each professional nurse will certainly have ideals and values on which she bases her own social actions, it is not her privilege to work for more widespread acceptance of her values through the use of her relations with patients. In this sphere each nurse may be informed on controversial issues but in relation to the patient's feelings about them *she is neutral, providing merely conditions and acting as a sounding board against which the patient may air his views and give full expression to his feelings in a nonjudgmental relationship.* It is distinctly unethical, in the traditional as well as the more modern sense, for a nurse to take advantage of a patient who is helpless and powerless. Undergoing a crisis that reinforces these feelings often demands clarification of the patient's own ethical principles and concepts; a professional nurse would not make use of his powerlessness to foster in him beliefs akin to her own.

Listening to a patient, watching for somatic responses, permitting the patient to have and to express his own feelings is a difficult task. It is easier to insinuate one's own thought and feelings upon the patient even though they are not useful to him. *The meaning of behavior of the patient to the pa-*

tient is the only relevant basis on which nurses can determine needs to be met. This is a simple matter when a mature patient expresses his needs verbally and when words correspond closely to the underlying feelings. More often than not

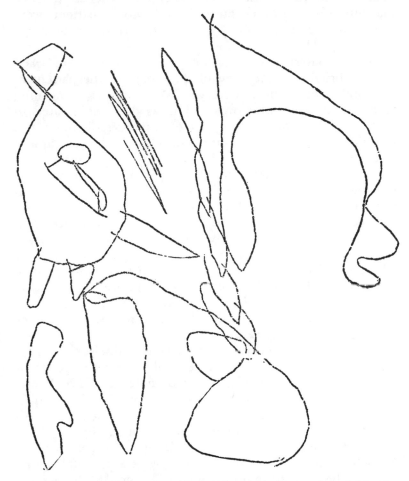

Fig. 12. A four-year-old child draws a picture in which she achieves unity of her father, mother, and herself, in a way in which it is not achieved in her present situation.

affectional, emotional needs are concealed and expressed in disguised ways. The difficulties in interpretation of the meaning of behavior are shown in Fig. 13, page 229. A group of students who were considering what is involved in everyday relationships with patients and the judgments in practice that nurses make in relation to the behavior of patients were given a simple pretest. They were asked to consider the drawings in Fig. 11, page 220 and Fig. 12, page 227, and to consider case materials as given on page 66. They were asked to state briefly the meaning of these data to the patient as interpreted by them as observers. Afterward, the meaning to the individuals who provided these data was related to them. Fig. 13 shows a sampling of responses obtained and the wide discrepancy between the meaning to the patient and to the observer.

The discrepancy between what a patient says about himself and what he does in relations with others is shown in the following example: Mr. White was a young father who entered the hospital with a diagnosis of duodenal ulcer that may require surgery. In conversation with nurses he speaks of his interest in youth movements, recreational activities for adolescents, and the importance and fun that he gets out of playing with his children and those in groups in which he spends his spare time. His conventional impression of himself is that of a pillar in the community and he wishes to convey this view to the nurses.

In the bed next to this patient is Jack, a nine-year-old boy, recovering from rheumatic fever. Observing the relations between these two patients it can be noted that Mr. White does not have genuine concern for the growth of the younger patient. His real interest is not in helping the boy in his struggle to construct a model airplane, but rather in showing the boy and the nurses how well he could make a plane himself. Instead of relating to the boy as a parental figure, who can be counted upon for help when needed, he is relating to him as another nine-year-old boy with whom he can compete on how well he can accomplish things, and thus gain

Fig. 12, p. 227	Fig. 11, p. 220	A Problem, case material, p. 66
"Trains and chickens. Destructive tendencies against object or individual."	"Hospital experience."	"Negative doctor suggestion."
"Child and mother going to trains to see chickens."	"Doctor wearing a mask." "Adjusting to fears."	"Insecurity. Adjusted to life crises then others called her attention to it."
"Someone is chasing him; his mother or teacher."	"Hospital experience." "Going somewhere happily and had an accident."	"Repressed fear."
"No love or affection has been given."	"Hospital scene."	"Doctor emphasized the psychic trauma too dramatically."
"Chickens on a railway."	"Shows adjustment to life—has had love and security but feels guilty."	"Doctors remarks changed her attitude."
"Loved one coming on a train and rejects killing chickens for food."		"Brooding and thinking makes one rebel."
"Creative aptitude."	"Accident and hospitalization."	"Fear of malignancy, cancer, and death."
"Going to church."		
"Drawing appears to be that of a four-year-old."	"Confusion of ideas."	"Attention focused on operation."
"Artist expresses own thoughts."	"Appears disoriented."	"Power of suggestion."
"Frustration—need for affection."	"A form of frustration caused this."	"Feeling different from others."
"Adult holding out arms."		"Retreating from reality."
"Holding out arms symbolic of: I want someone to take me."	"Ideal of self as normal but personality disorganized."	"Feels more alone and needs affection."
"Child making drawing of his toys and animals."	"No special meaning."	"Too introverted."
"A great deal of force."	"A very confused mind."	"Too few hobbies."
"Looks like usual attempts of four-year-olds."	"Various elements that are giving trouble."	"Neurotic because of physician's suggestion."

Fig. 13. A sampling of responses of twenty-one students to a simple pretest on the meaning of behavior to the patient, as recognized by the observer.

the approval of the nurses. Unless the nurse is aware of this need, that apparently was unmet in his own earlier experiences, she cannot help the nine-year-old patient to gain the satisfaction of constructing an airplane himself. Nor can she relate helpfully to the patient who is chronologically older unless she takes into account his needs to experience and to complete being a juvenile.

The nurse can help the older patient by aiding him to become aware of his personal needs projected into the younger patient's activities. Without showing approval or disapproval she could say, "You would enjoy struggling to build an airplane, too, but Jack will learn by doing it himself. Perhaps we could ask your family to bring in something that you could construct that would interest you."

Another illustration points to the operation of a patient's concept of self as one who waits for others to give her approval and whatever is needed. Barbara is fifteen years old. Although all of the nurses like her, she asserts that she is a hypocrite because she would like to be a nurse, too, but becomes annoyed when other patients fuss a great deal about their pain. She is somewhat of a martyr about her own, not admitting that she has pain unless it is unusually severe. She tries constantly to please everyone—her mother, father, friends, and the nurses. She thinks the nurses consider her a fake because she doesn't get out of bed and do things for herself, although there is no order for her to be out of bed. She makes no demands upon nurses but rather waits until the last minute and then requests something that must be given to her immediately—such as a bedpan. She remarks frequently about the beauty of others in the situation, but has not in any way expressed her feelings about herself and the rather extensive contractions that she has as a result of severe burns.

Why does Barbara tell the nurses that she is a hypocrite? Is it so that she can hear them say, again and again, "But, Barbara, you aren't." Is this a way of constantly reassuring herself of and feeling secure in their approval? What might happen if the nurses said, "You feel that you are a hypocrite because you don't like to hear other patients make demands upon nurses"? This remark, which shows neither approval nor disapproval, requires Barbara to re-examine her remark if she wishes to make another comment. Reassuring her that she is not a hypocrite does not help her to expand why she thinks so. Her expectations that others expect her to do more than she can do while in bed show both her view of self and her view of others. At some time she has been made to feel that she was a fake, if she could not perform beyond the circumstances of the situation and she entertains expectations that the nurses view her in the same light, although none of them have said this directly to her. Barbara's need to be liked by everyone, and her unconditional relations with others in order to achieve their approval, is a negative way of gaining enhancement of her view of self which is quite shallow. Everyone has the right to expect and to receive assistance from nurses when they need it in a situation in which nurses operate. Why does Barbara feel that she must strive so hard to make sure that she can timidly permit this right to be expressed?

Another experience with a patient, described by a nurse, gives clues to the concept of self that operates in the relationship. Miss Way was forty-eight years old and had been crippled as a result of polio which she suffered at the age of three years. She had been in and out of the hospital several times for rather vague illnesses but this time she had a fractured femur. Very soon after admission she had her radio, her pillow, her hot plate, and daily meals sent in from home, and was sure to give the nurses specific directions on how she wanted these possessions used. When she suffered severe pain she expected the whole ward full of patients to be quiet; when she felt comfortable she found great pleasure in making fun of other patients. She had many complaints including chronic constipation.

When the patient's mother visited it could be noted that she was a most meticulous woman. She frequently talked about what a "good, well-trained, and beautiful child" the patient had been before the bout with poliomyelitis. After this serious illness she had one treatment after another, growing more and more deformed, and apparently, from her mother's comments, more and more rejected by her mother who felt it her duty to continue to care for her in an unconditional way. It can be speculated that at a very early age this child realized her opportunity to exert power over her mother which may not have been respected before her illness. She constantly tried to give the nurses gifts and when they took them would say, "I don't know why those nurses don't like me, I gave them such nice things."

Any disabling disease is perceived as an interference to ongoing development. Any threat to the self requires a defense. It is hard to say what this patient's concept of self was like at age three but if her mother has constantly reminded everyone how "good, well-trained, and beautiful" she was, it is easy to see how this patient has become the person she is because she felt that she could not live up to her mother's lost expectations and at the same time have the security of mother love when she needed it most. That she has become a passive and more or less biting kind of person, as a way of defending herself against feelings of helplessness seems obvious.

What can a nurse hope to accomplish after forty-five years of domination of her mother? Rather than comment approvingly or disapprovingly on the requests and the food that is brought in, could the nurse say rather simply, "You prefer your own pillow to the ones the hospital can supply," or, "You prefer to have your mother prepare your food to what we serve here," or, "You prefer to have the ward quiet because you are feeling pain." When the patient makes biting comments about other patients, these too can be reflected back as a way of helping the patient to become more aware of what she is saying. Depriving the patient of the services she demands is likely to make her more demanding and more defensive; helping her to become aware of what is involved in her demands and her comments, in a way that does not stamp them as good or bad, aids the patient to take cognizance of her feelings and their relation to her present predicament. When a patient is aided in a way that puts the lead in the patient's hands, allowing feelings to be expressed as and when the patient is ready to express them, it is less likely to lead to the development of severe anxiety.

A nonproductive orientation toward life and a constricted view of self do not necessarily mean that a patient cannot work and become successful in conventional terms.[10] It means that his relations with others are not creative in terms of the growth and personality development of himself and others. Mr. Grove, a man who was very much concerned about his health all of his life, illustrates this point. His mother had tuberculosis and he always felt that she should not have had children; his fear of the disease and the rejection by her that he felt on being separated from her early in life led to overconcern for health that was not justified in his health history.

Everything that Mr. Grove did in life centered around his health needs. He wrote a book that elaborated his private concerns. He owned a large and thriving business in one state and then decided that the climate was not too good for his health. He moved to another state and again purchased a business that met with considerable financial success. These riches made it possible for him to have his meals especially prepared in accordance with his health needs. If he went out for an evening of entertainment, and then discovered that it would tax him too much, he would leave and return home. He finally gave up going to church because it was too drafty. Despite all of these conditions that he placed upon living, he managed to raise a family and to amass a considerable fortune. His concept of himself as an ill person governed his life. His relations with others were meager, based on the feeling that he had only so much health and strength to expend in life and that this had to be conserved.

Mr. Smythe has been hospitalized for a number of years

[10] Fromm, *op. cit.*

with paraplegia. He is neat, clean, and very exacting about all of his personal effects. Usually he is quiet and unfriendly with others. He is very critical of the hospital when talking with patients, particularly when a nurse is within hearing distance, but he does not communicate his complaints directly to the nurses. He sets himself apart from other patients and refuses to eat in the dining room, although he is able to get around in his wheel chair. A special tray is brought to him when other bedfast patients are fed. This has been the patient's pattern for several years.

Recently a nurse brought a tray, prepared by the dietitian, and offered it to the patient. The patient looked at it and said, "You can give that slop to the pigs, I won't touch it." The nurse responded, taking the tray away, "Very well, it is what the dietitian prepared." While the nurse in question was feeding other patients another nurse appeared on the scene. Without knowing what had transpired previously between the patient and the first nurse, the second nurse picked up the tray and placed it before him. The patient ate parts of it without further comment.

This case material serves to illustrates the momentary nature of responses and the possibility of the discharge of a hostile feeling leading to a less hostile one. If the first nurse had communicated to the second that the patient had refused the tray, and that there was no point in serving it again, the patient's wish to eat that had emerged after his hostility was expressed could not have found satisfaction. It is difficult to accept a patient as he is when his hostility is constantly expressed, seemingly in order to sever his relations with others. Actually, the hostility serves to protect the patient against further threats to his personality. *The situation is not hopeless until nurses in the situation think it is, for they will then relate to the patient in ways that communicate to him their inability to accept him as a person despite his hostile feelings.* This patient seems to be focusing on behavior that will bring him disapproval, perhaps because he cannot tolerate approval that is shown him for his interest in books and his accomplishments in occupational therapy. Until his feelings about his illness, and its meaning to him is clear to him and to the nurses who take care of him, communication will be governed by the autistic meaning of events as seen by nurses and the patient.

Praise, blame, indifference, and learning in nursing situations

Praising the patient is often thought to be one of the more effectual ways to encourage the patient to take an interest in his present surroundings. Blaming the patient is taboo in nursing, so it rarely can be observed directly as an aspect of the face-to-face nurse-patient relationship. Indifference toward a patient is held excusable on the grounds that nurses are very busy. It might be well to consider here what is accomplished by these methods and how these outcomes are different from those achieved when a nurse aids the patient to focus upon learning.

A patient in a hospital situation is always more or less powerless. One of the unique differences in hospital and public health nursing may be the fact that a patient in his own home has relatively greater power than does the hospitalized patient. It is the relationship of individual power to the power asserted by authorities in situations that requires understanding by a nurse who wishes to aid patients to grow. Nurses have rational power in the knowledge of their profession; they are not entitled to irrational power over individuals, such as may often be inferred in conditional relations, i.e., "I will accept you as a patient if you do this and that." Yet praise or indifference are often used as authority by indirection and thus as coercions to get the patient to do something that he does not understand as necessary or desirable.

Praising a patient is always conditioned by the nurse's need to give praise. In a patient who has adapted all of his behavior in the direction of getting approval of others, regardless of the merits of what is being approved, praise closes off the possibilities of learning and it arouses greater ambition, competitiveness, and feelings of superiority. The patient then behaves in terms of what brings praise. Interpersonal relations may generate anxiety so that the patient must focus almost exclusively on what the nurse is willing to praise, rather than focusing on what is desirable learning in relation to his problem.

Focusing on the learning requires that the nurse will be able to help the patient to identify next steps in the problem. It depends upon a deeply felt respect for each individual and his capacities and his right to use them to accomplish what he can. It depends upon her recognition that the patient can undergo productive experiences which will grow as he comes to recognize for himself what he is able to do.

In some patients, those with cerebral palsy for instance, any pressure may give rise to anxiety that defeats learning. For example, a particular patient was doing exceptionally well in learning how to handle her difficulties in motor co-ordination. Following an experience in a hospital, she was not able to continue learning as she had done before. No reason could be found for this interference with previously adequate learning. When nurses who cared for her in the hospital were asked to confer with clinic authorities it was discovered that they had given the girl a great deal of praise during her hospital stay. It is well known that the patient with cerebral palsy disorganizes quickly under any kind of tension, pressure, or urgency. Praise in this instance was looked upon as pressure to do better than she could anticipate; it was blame by implication and each time she set out to focus on learning she could recall the flowery praise to which she was expected to live up in the present situation.

When a patient accomplishes something that is a fact, a nurse can say so. For example, "You walked the length of the hall this morning for the first time." To add, "That is wonderful," may raise doubts in the mind of the patient and close off the learning that is possible for him. Or, it may make it necessary for him to overdo, walking up and down the corridor until he is fatigued, in order to get more praise than some other patient.

Praise and blame, good and bad, right and wrong, leave nurses only a two-sided coin with which to operate in their relations with patients. Focusing on the steps in learning allows infinite variety in relations with patients and may contribute something worthwhile to the general level of growth in present-day civilization.

Summary

One of the most important tasks in life is that of identifying oneself. A concept of self does not form and then operate once and for all; each recurring problem challenges the view of self that an individual holds and demands defenses of it or permits further expansion. The patient's total personality focuses on each difficulty that arises as a medical problem is faced with professional help. The patient comes to understand the nurse's personality through her attitudes and assistance given in relation to a problem. In order to understand the concept of self held by a nurse and a patient it is necessary to look back upon child-rearing patterns and the situations in which discovery of self was permitted or not. Problems that arise when this task is not successfully accomplished arise when there is a clash between the patient's expectations of the nurse and the nurse's view of a patient. A nurse cannot be flexible in her relations with all patients unless she has examined the basis within herself that makes it possible for her to accept all patients as they are. The patient and nurse views of self are not automatically compatible. Permitting the patient to count upon the nurse for help often requires unconditional acceptance of the patient, as well as alertness to cues to growth and to the wish to be independent of the nurse's help. The nurse who cannot vary her roles as she observes what is happening in an evolving relationship may keep a patient anchored at a level of dependence or urge him too fast in the direction of independence. As the nurse and patient come to know and to respect each other, as they work out ways of focusing on the patient's difficulties in a common struggle, an interdependent relationship with one another develops. Each individual becomes a person to the degree that a whole concept of self makes possible interdependent relations with others that are productive for all. While the interaction of adults with the growing child lays the foundation for a concept of self, succeeding experiences can reinforce positive traits and aid in the modification of negative views of self.

CHAPTER **11**

Developing Skills in Participation

Overview

A DEMOCRATIC SOCIETY requires participation of all members. Deliberation and discussion of problems leads to understanding of the problem and of the evidence on which decisions can be based. When all members participate in making decisions that affect them, they are more likely to understand what is involved in the goals they have chosen. Involvement in the process of setting goals that affect oneself as a member of a group builds respect for the integrity of other individuals as the opinions and attitudes of each are evaluated and reshaped as a plan for meeting the needs of all is designed.

When an individual faces a medical problem there is merit in securing his participation in setting new goals and in planning activities or experiences that seem likely to lead to a workable solution to the problem. Nurses cannot teach solutions to problems that will be useful to every patient. Patients can be aided to experience the steps in attacking a problem and develop skills required for participating in its solution. The development of skills in participation is a fourth psychological task, which builds upon the three tasks already discussed. In this chapter, information on the development of skills in participation will be given and will be related to problems that arise in situations in which nurses practice.

239

Essential questions

Who should tell the patient about his medical problem? How much should a patient be permitted to know about his problem? Can a nurse secure co-operation from a patient without his understanding what is involved in his problem? Can a patient act upon solutions to his problem advised by others without recognizing and comprehending the problem? Can nursing function as an instrument that is therapeutic and educative for patients when it teaches solutions to problems? What do patients learn when a nurse tells them what must be done? What do patients learn when they are aided to look at the evidence and to arrive at a decision on what might be done?

How does learning take place in individuals? Should nurses take into account the process of learning, in their relations with patients? Isn't it simpler to let the physician prescribe and carry out what is ordered? Patients can be told, simply, "Your doctor ordered it." What are the obligations to society that a nurse needs to consider: to get the patient out of the hospital as quickly as possible in whatever way seems most direct or to help patients to use experiences such as illness as steppingstones for further development of personality? Who should decide what a nurse should do in relation to the patient's ability to participate or his lacks in skills required for building a democratic society?

These questions when discussed in professional groups are likely to bring into focus many issues concerning interprofessional relations. Assumptions that guide professional relations with patients and policies that nourish the growth of professional persons and patients can grow out of discussion of these questions. They all hinge, more or less, around the question: should the patient participate in understanding and solving his problem, or should he be a passive receptor of medical advice and solutions?

Personality formation in childhood: background information

In order to understand the dynamics of interpersonal relations in a sickroom, or in a patient's home, or in a clinic, where a nurse and patient come together, it is helpful to look at genetically older experiences and to gather clues from past development. Methods for defending oneself during illness, and for coping with threats to personality and to a view of self that is held may be inappropriate in the current situation. However, in past experiences these methods seemed to work and to provide the individual with a measure of safety at a time when he was feeling anxious, insecure, and powerless. It is helpful to examine experiences in childhood in order to determine when participation is possible for a child, and the way in which skills for co-operating with others are learned.

Sullivan characterizes the "eras" of personality development in somewhat different fashion from other workers in the field.[1] During the "juvenile era," which occurs roughly between the ages of six and nine, several important abilities begin to develop in relations with other children of the same age and interests. The capacity to arbitrate, to reach consent in a group by making individual concessions that are mutually agreed upon, a capacity that Sullivan refers to as *"compromise"* ripens during this era. The ability to struggle with others of the same age, to express open rivalry for an object or a position in the group, develops at this age; Sullivan calls this a capacity for *"competition."* The ability of a number of individuals to subordinate personal wishes in order to derive mutual benefit and to identify shared goals, is a third capacity which Sullivan refers to as *"co-operation."*

The evolution of capacities for co-operation, competition, and compromise is basic to skill in participating collaboratively with others in a democratic society and in the solution of personal problems. Many adults seem to think that a child

[1] H. S. Sullivan, *op. cit.;* Patrick Mullahy, *Oedipus: Myth and Complex* (New York, Hermitage House, Inc., 1948), pp. 301-07.

is capable of developing and using these abilities earlier in life. Indeed, in groups of children playing together, in a park or in a nursery school, it often looks as if these abilities were already in operation. However, closer observation shows each child to be egocentric and autistic in his behavior; when co-operation seems to be observed it is momentary, unsustained, and sometimes in compliance with the wishes of the adults who are present and upon whom the child is dependent for approval.

During these three years, from ages six to nine, children in groups begin more and more to demand the use of these abilities from their companions. These are the methods that work in the group. Other methods, such as whining, crying, demanding, may work at home or with other adults but in the group of children they are inacceptable. Children who use these earlier methods for meeting their needs are viewed as different from the gang and are often ostracized for their lacks in skill. A child who has been able to use relations with his parents to talk things over and to express his feelings without being deprived of the need to communicate honestly will be ready to move on to these experiences and will readily develop these emergent abilities further in a group made up of children of his own age. Children who cannot profit by and learn from these experiences are hampered by their expectations, and by their perceptions of the new experience in a genetically older way. Children who have given up the wish to struggle, the wish to produce and to contribute, the wish to express themselves and to undergo the risks involved in inquiring, cannot move on to a wish to participate with their peers. Longings, unfulfilled wishes, and desires becloud their perception of the new experience; they are likely to view it as one in which their older wishes and longings will be fulfilled rather than one in which new desires can be explored.

Observation in nursery schools often shows children acting out genetically older wishes. One little girl age seven will continually try to "mother" another child, selecting one with whom she can act out her conception of a good mother and at the same time review her own mother's domination over her. The other little girl, accustomed to being dominated by stronger individuals, permits full regimentation of what she may do in the dramatic play. Other children cannot enter into spontaneous play since in earlier experiences their spontaneity was quickly checked and ruled out as undesirable behavior in the company of adults. A child who shows rage at home, when her wishes are frustrated and when she finds it difficult to comply with demands of adults that seem unreasonable to her, is told that her behavior "is not nice." Yet, rage is a spontaneous response which from the child's perception of a situation is justified. It is the child's way of responding to a perception of disapproval and disrespect for the child's own capacities to feel and to act in her own behalf.

Children who have not been permitted to contribute their ideas and feelings and have them accepted and acted upon wisely cannot feel free to put their ideas into the market place of free competition of ideas as it is developed by a group of seven-year-olds. In their past experience the method that worked was compliance with ideas and feelings posed as acceptable and "right" by adults, and they feel safe only when they adhere to what is approved by individuals who have made their power over them felt in telling ways.

The earlier appraisals of a child, made by parents, carry over into later situations. "Johnny is a naughty boy; Mother doesn't like Johnny when he is naughty" when repeated as a chronic suggestion on how mother views Johnny may be taken into the child's perception of himself and become his view of self. Appropriate naughty actions then are used to live out this view of self. Or, a mother may say, "Mary, I want you to stay clean. You are a good girl and I don't want you to get dirty like those other children." When Mary's group decided to wear dungarees and to build a tremendous tunnel out of wet sand Mary cannot join them; she is held back by her mother's expectations of her and her need for approval from adults. A mother might repeatedly assert to her child, "I don't want you to play with that gang. They are ruffians.

You will get hurt and I don't want you to get hurt." Again, the child is prevented from taking all of the risks that are involved in playing with a group of children her own age and at the same time developing the abilities necessary for future participation in life in a productive way. Her participation is more likely to be that of a passive receptor, accepting what others say is "right," devoting her time to reading and studying without making these hours of inquiry count in later social relations, seeking approval in being "right" rather than satisfaction in contributing to the development of a society in which all are interrelated, interdependent, a universe of discourse.

When a child has not identified himself in an affirmative way, earlier processes are reinforced and newer processes cannot be utilized. An infant uses *empathy,* that is, he observes what others feel about him and identifies his feelings about the world in terms of the feelings of others. An infant and growing child may comply with demands that others make upon him but at the same time use his imagination to invent highly personal or *autistic* meanings for what is being experienced. Autism is characterized by references to the self, rather than to the reality situation as a group might see it. Children use first the *cry* then *speech* to communicate their wants and needs, but when these communications are persistently viewed as inacceptable to adults the child may learn to use these same tools to distort communication, to prevent others from finding out what is wanted. While this distortion is highly developed, and can be observed in extreme degrees in patients diagnosed as schizophrenic, it can also be observed in everyday communications. The person who makes a derogatory remark and then says, "I am sorry," is using speech to achieve satisfaction in expressing hostility and to amend it. The person who stalls, who resists committing himself before a group, who impedes progress in discussion by getting away from the point and then says, "Perhaps I shouldn't have brought this up," is also an individual who rarely views himself as a person who wishes to delay progress in communication. These ways of entering into the work of a group are ways that worked in earlier years when the child's ability to see clearly and to come to the point directly were not permitted, and disrespect for the child as a person was shown. The child's power is then put to use through the tools available to him in a way that ensures feelings of safety.

Following the juvenile era, Sullivan identifies an epoch called "preadolescence." [2] During this period the abilities that were exercised earlier are more or less consolidated and the child strengthens skills in participation by learning to use a process Sullivan calls "consensual validation." The capacity for making use of this process ripens between the ages of eight and one-half and twelve, roughly speaking. Validation by consensus is a social experience through which a child comes to see himself more or less as his chums view him. Autistic conceptions of self are shed as the youth expresses himself— his feeling and ideas—freely and compares data with others in the group. In this experience of sharing views, talking it over with youth of approximately the same age and the same sex, a reorganization of previous experience takes place and a realistic view of life and the world, and one's role in it, emerges.

According to Sullivan, the capacity for love is released during this period of growing up. We have already defined mother love as unconditional, as the ability to accept the child as he is, whatever his constitutional inheritance and expression—in terms of physique, intelligence, and temperament. That is, *mother love* is the capacity to love one's child as he is, for being himself, for expressing his feelings and ideas as they are felt rather than as adults would prefer them to be. In contrast, *love,* as it operates between people other than mother and child, requires the ability to care for and accept others as much as one cares for and accepts the self.[3, 4] Not

[2] Sullivan, *op. cit.;* Mullahy, *op. cit.,* p. 308.
[3] Sullivan, *op. cit.;* Mullahy, *op. cit.,* p. 307.
[4] Erich Fromm, *Man for Himself* (New York, Rinehart & Company, Inc., 1947).

more, not less, but to the extent that one appreciates oneself can the capacity to love others be felt and expressed.

Up until the age of eight and one-half the child has been largely concerned with adapting himself to the demands of others and with gaining skills required for living. When adaptations and skills have been acquired in a way that does not require denial of self, ability to consider the needs of others can appear during preadolescence. At this time, chums of the same sex talk over their most intimate feelings about people and sympathy for the feelings of others develops. These relationships between two boys or two girls are often thought of as homosexual leanings but Sullivan points out that homosexuality occurs when there is inability to move from this stage in development toward heterosexual relations during adolescence.[5]

The reasons why some youths cannot move forward may be found in present and past experiences. How a mother feels about her daughter or son confiding in a chum and not in her makes a difference. How the youth feels about sustaining his mother's or father's approval at this point makes a difference. The skills that each youth has for developing a chum relationship aids the process of validating experiences and arriving at views of the self and the world that are realistic in terms of opportunity, level of aspiration, and inherent capacities—all have a bearing on the successful outcome of learning during this period.

When a youth has successfully undergone all of the experiences discussed so far and developed skill in participating actively with others in designing one's role in life, as a step toward redesigning the society in which one lives, he is ready to meet crises that arise during adolescence. The reawakening of sexual drives and hormonal changes that take place in the body lead to emergence of the "lust dynamism," as Sullivan calls it.[6]

Skills for living competently in a rapidly changing world

[5] Sullivan, *op. cit.*; Mullahy, *op. cit.*, pp. 307-08.
[6] Mullahy, *op. cit.*, pp. 308-11.

are developed step by step as the infant progresses through childhood into adolescence and toward maturity. Failure to develop skills at any point leads to incompetence in participation in dealing with recurring problems in life. Ineffective participation in life impedes the development of a democratic society in which all are free to grow, to change, to mature, and to design a way of life that ensures productive relations among people.

Skills in participation as required in nursing situations

Nurses aid patients who have varying degrees of skill in meeting the problems in life that recur and that affect the health of individuals and their communities. In this work, we would like to base discussion of problems in nursing on the assumption that the nurse has a responsibility to aid patients in improving their skills in meeting problems rather than in teaching solutions to problems.

The patient's way of viewing his problem is governed by the concept of self that he holds and the skills that he has available for tackling the tasks at hand. Any situation that generates concern, in the nurse or patient, calls out the available resources in those individuals in process of meeting the situation. The first step in solving a problem is identifying the difficulty.

Any medical problem usually gives rise to many related difficulties. Thus, a patient whose major problem is that of recovering from a broken leg and resuming his obligations in a family and a community will face a number of difficulties that constitute the total problem. They are often expressed rather simply, "Will I walk again," "When will my leg stop hurting," "I can't sleep," "Food doesn't taste good to me here and I can't eat." Nurse and patient together tackle each one of these difficulties as they arise; meeting each one successfully and educatively for the patient leads to the solution of the larger problem. For example, the patient says, "I can't sleep." He has *identified a subproblem*. A nurse might repeat, "You can't sleep. I wonder what some of the reasons might be." That is, she helps the patient to *gather evidence* pertinent to understanding the problem. The patient might respond, "Well, this bed is too hard; I'm used to two pillows instead of one; I'm used to getting a lot of exercise; I'm a pretty active person in my work; I keep thinking about lots of things just as I'm ready to fall off to sleep." The nurse might respond, "I wonder what we could do about each of those items." They might decide to tackle the bed and pillow difficulty first. The patient and nurse can then discuss what is possible in the particular hospital and situation in which the patient finds himself. Together, they can achieve a decision on what is possible, what can be done, and then move on to other items that have been mentioned and other *possible courses of action* that can be taken in behalf of and with the co-operation of the patient. They can decide to *try out what is proposed*, concerning rearrangement of the bed and pillows for example, the nurse suggesting, "Let's try this tonight, and tomorrow you can let me know whether we should take another look at the difficulty and decide to try something else."

In considering a difficulty in the manner described the patient is permitted to use his capacities and to improve his skill in tackling problems. Emphasis is placed on what both can decide together, in full consideration of what is possible in a particular hospital, rather than upon the patient putting up with the problem until he gets home where he can solve it in his own way. This is a way of helping patients to develop skill in participating with others in reaching and abiding by decisions that affect them. When the procedure described is followed what does the patient learn? Does he learn that nurses appreciate difficulties that he has to face, that they are willing to expend effort to help him to face problems, that they will not rob him of his own powers to contribute to the illumination of the problem and the development of courses of action, and that they are genuinely concerned with his welfare? Under what circumstances does the patient learn that nurses have "stock phrases" and "pat answers" that are used in robot fashion and that convey the impression that the patient's difficulties are too minor to be given any kind of consideration?

The way in which a patient views the problem determines how he will act in attempting to solve it. Attitudes of the patient are made up of needs and feelings, or emotions; in order to aid a patient toward understanding a problem it is necessary to permit the patient to reveal in his own words how he feels about the problem.[7] Attitudes are interlocked with the patient's communications, verbal and nonverbal, as the difficulty is phrased for the nurse. As the patient is able to reveal his genuine attitudes to himself, and to a nurse as a sounding board against which he can reflect what he says and feels, he can become aware of his attitudes and thus expand his understanding of a problem. Involvement of the self in the problem precedes expansion of what is understood about it. The patient's first whole impression of the problem may be inadequate, may not indicate to him all that is involved.[8] Or the patient may be overconcerned with a few of the details and become lost in grappling with them before all of the steps in the whole problem are clearly seen. Or, the patient may be seeking a quick solution, as a way of relieving anxiety, and as a way of avoiding responsibility involved in seeing the whole problem.

Assisting a patient to formulate and to attack a central, all-pervasive problem in interpersonal relations is the task of a competent psychiatrist. But, the operations in the uncovering processes are the same, basically, whether the problem at hand is a revision of a nursing procedure, the development of a solution to rivalry among a group of patients in a public, general hospital, or the uncovering of the central difficulty of the analysand by a psychoanalyst working together with his pa-

[7] David Kretch and Richard S. Crutchfield, *Theory and Problems of Social Psychology* (New York, McGraw-Hill Book Company, Inc., 1948), pp. 254-55. See also, M. Sherif and H. Cantril, *The Psychology of Ego-involvements* (New York, John Wiley & Sons, Inc., 1947).

[8] Max Wertheimer, *Productive Thinking* (New York, Harper & Brothers, 1945), p. 191.

tient. A nurse who helps a patient to grapple with a difficulty stated as, "I can't sleep," uses the same steps but not the same depth in this problem that an analyst or a scientist of any kind uses in reaching a solution to another problem.

In general, when the problem has to do with *things*—as in the standardization of a procedure—consideration of the problems involved can be arbitrarily limited by the time factor that is known to operate in advance. In the field of behavior, where the problems have to do with human *forces* that are personal and social, nurses must again consider the time factor. An analysand can arrange for long term consideration of a central problem in advance, and the analyst can be guided by the time that will be available for the work that is necessary. A nurse cannot be assured that a problem will be worked through and must therefore *permit the lead to come from the patient,* at his own rate of interest and speed, as he permits her to listen to his feelings and his difficulties in relations with people. A patient will generally go only as far as it is safe for him to go, in getting a clearer view of his difficulty. When time functions as a coercion for the nurse, and she attempts premature solution to the patient's problem by "telling" the patient what is wrong and what must be done about his feelings or informing him on the meaning of his feelings, as she understands them, she is likely to do damage to the patient. More often than not, crucial interpersonal problems are not recognized and not infrequently the *symptoms* are thought to be the problem, although they are merely aspects of expression of the problem rather than the crucial difficulty itself.

This is well borne out in the symptom of thumb sucking, as so frequently seen in children. Pediatricians point out that thumb sucking is a sign that shows that an underlying need of the child is not being met; the problem is the identification and satisfaction of that need. To strap the child's thumb and to pour foul tasting medicines on it is to do violence to the child's personality.

It is primarily for this reason that advice and suggestion, in the areas of feelings and emotions, are not thought to be useful and are not advised in this work. In an interpersonal situation where there is a notable problem in relatedness to people, it is likely that the patient has had advice, reassurance, or suggestions in many forms through his friends, family, work associates, press and radio. These forms of advice are rarely taken into account, they do not aid patients to bring about significant changes in a way of living except in ways that are often harmful. If the matter were simply one of telling patients what is wrong with their feelings, reminding them of their interpersonal problems, most—if not all—of the psychiatric patients in psychiatric institutions would probably be well, for they have all had much advice in similar fashion.

The processes for recognition and solution of a problem, like the processes of self-renewal, self-repair, self-awareness, arise within the individual. Behavior that is purposeful and productive is made possible by these processes and must be initiated by the self of the doer. Interpersonal conditions in the situation can be improved so that the responding patient will want to reveal his *problems to himself;* the question is not one of revealing the problem to give information to others but rather so that what has been discovered can be acted upon in awareness without suppression and distortion. As Wertheimer has pointed out so clearly, the patient learns only as he re-creates the steps, re-experiences the feelings, and views them in a new perspective.[9] This is possible when significant help is available. Nursing process and method offer significant help.

A conversation between an auxiliary worker and a personnel worker in a hospital illustrates failure to identify the problem:

Auxiliary worker:	*Personnel worker:*
"Good morning, Miss Howe" (spoken with effort).	"Good morning, Jane. It is 7:20 A.M. and you know you *should* be here on time especially with the schedule of work we have today" (spoken with annoyance).

[9] *Ibid.*

Auxiliary worker:

"I just can't seem to make it. I get up at 6:30 but I have too much to do" (spoken with effort).

One hour later:

"Yes, Miss Howe" (spoken faintly).

"I went to breakfast" (expressed haughtily).

"Miss Howe, I've wanted to talk to you for a long time. Please don't tell me what to do. After all, you aren't the supervisor. If I want to come on late I will" (spoken with derision). (Note how she has caught on to the value of "please," as a prelude to a derogatory remark.)

Personnel worker:

"Well, Jane, *I* think you could make a little more effort to be on time. You live right here and you really haven't any excuse" (spoken with some annoyance).

"Jane."
"Jane, where were you? *I needed* you to fix something and you weren't around" (expressed with some exaggeration).
"Please let some one know the next time you leave here. No one knew where you were. You *should* have had your breakfast before you came to work" (annoyance becoming more pronounced).

(Immediately on guard) "Jane, I may not be the supervisor but at this moment *I'm in charge* of getting this work done. *I* can't have things running smoothly unless people come on time and work together. Something will have to be done about this situation."

While this personnel worker finally asserts that there is need to work together, it can be seen from the data that her own highly personal needs and goals are not conducive to achievement of participation. The auxiliary worker posed her problem very early in the conversation, saying, "I have too much to do." Inquiring into what is involved in this problem and working out a course of action that would be useful for Jane and for the work situation might have led to a more fruitful outcome for all concerned. Since there was no personal warmth, no human relatedness between these two people, Jane could not take in and respond to all of the "I needed" and "shoulds" of Miss Howe; her own difficulties and needs took precedence and she responded in terms of satisfying them. *Participation among workers requires human interest in and respect for each as a person and an opportunity to explore personal needs and ways in which they may be met to the satisfaction of all.* What is needed on the job cannot be communicated until there is mutual respect and the job is viewed as a common goal.

The following experience shows a nurse aiding a patient to identify a problem and to base his course of action on available evidence:

Patient:

Mr. Boone, a sixty-five-year-old farmer, came to X Sanitarium with a note stating that he should be admitted as soon as possible for treatment of moderately advanced tuberculosis. He was told that he would be notified when a bed was available. The staff member who interviewed him seemed unable to find out Mr. Boone's correct address; because he could not communicate this clearly and since he needed supervision until admission to the sanitarium was possible, a nurse was sent out to make a home visit.

"Well, that nurse down there at X Sanitarium told me that it would be several weeks before I could come in so I have just come home from Y Sanitarium. I am trying to get in there right away. I have lived in X county all my life, except when we go down to Y county for a few months in the

Nurse:

On arrival the nurse said, "Since there is going to be quite a long wait before you can be admitted to X Sanitarium I thought I would visit and see if you have any questions about carrying on your treatment at home."

Patient: *Nurse:*

summertime. I went to X Sanitarium because that is where my doctor sent me and that is where I thought I belonged. I have paid taxes in X county all my life. I am willing to pay. I don't want charity. I only want what I am entitled to."

"You are right. You wouldn't be accepting charity in X Sanitarium; it is there for the people in X county to use when they need it. If you have lived in X county for the last eight years you are certainly entitled to be admitted there as soon as there is a bed for you."

(To his wife) "Mary, you go in and get those tax receipts."

"Now here are the receipts for the last twenty years. We have lived here for that long. We were staying in Y county when I got sick and I guess that is how I got mixed up when I talked to the lady at the Sanitarium. I gave that address instead of this one."

"You have established that you live in X county."

"Now, Nurse, I want you to tell me honestly, what shall I do? Shall I go over to Y county and get into the hospital right away or shall I wait to get into X Sanitarium?"

"Then I will wait. What can I do while I am at home?"

"I guess you have established the county in which you are entitled to use the hospital."

It is noteworthy in the foregoing material that as the patient was able to visualize all that was legally involved in making a decision on where to be hospitalized, through his own evidence largely, he was able to choose a useful course of action. Following this choice, a new problem emerged and he was able to turn to the nurse who respected his ability to decide wisely and seek further help from her. As these superficial difficulties are cleared up he may get to his feelings about having tuberculosis and he will have developed some skills for reaching an understanding of what is involved.

An illustration of a way in which a nurse might aid a patient to develop the wish to participate is given in the following incident: A very wealthy woman, a socialite and daughter-in-law of a prominent physician, is admitted to the maternity floor of a hospital. Upon admission, she attempts to impress all hospital personnel with her importance and at the same time complains about everything that is done. The patient uses abusive and profane language. As the delivery room nurse comes to visit her in her room, she discovers the patient calling her father-in-law and asking him to "come at once and tell these people what to do." Her husband and mother stand by, apparently immobilized by these performances that cannot be understood immediately. On examination the nurse finds that the stage of labor requires transferring her to the labor room. There the patient continues to yell, scream, curse, and complain; her efforts are so involved in these activities that she cannot co-operate with the nurse or with the physiological processes that are to aid in the delivery of her child.

A nurse would have to be quite clear about her preconceptions about people who come from certain social classes and about how women in labor *should* behave. If she starts with the premise that *each patient will behave, during any crisis, in a way that has worked in relation to crises faced in the past,* the nurse has made a head start on accepting this patient as she is. Knowing the expected roles patients from various economic groupings feel they should play, would clarify what is going on. If the nurse can come to appreciate that this method of relating to strangers, when facing a new experience that is not clearly visualized, is one that is more likely to incur contempt and dislike in others, and thus to get them to take aggressive action against the patient that will justify expectations that the patient holds for some valid reason, she will have taken the second step toward accepting the patient as she is. In the case material cited the nurse merely delivered the baby, in the absence of the physician, in a way that would protect the baby and prevent tearing the patient's perineum. These technical skills can be used in a matter of fact manner that permits the patient to feel what she needs to feel at this particular time. When a nurse has an opportunity to prepare a patient psychologically for delivery, which was not possible in this event, it is useful to help the patient to review her feelings and her expectations about what is about to take place. When a patient is hyperactive and showing overconcern for her own safety, the patient's feelings can be discussed with greater clarity after the event has been undergone.

There are probably many reasons why this patient could not co-operate; one can speculate that skill in participation was not learned earlier in life and put to use in meeting crises that demanded revisions in her concept of self. The meaning of the pattern of behavior used can be revealed only by the patient, but a nurse who is aware of her own feelings and secure in her professional skills can withstand these kinds of relationships and wait for an appropriate time to aid the patient to view her problem.

The nurse who documented the experience cited had many mixed feelings at the time; however, she was so busy with delivering the baby that she was unable to act upon them. She felt that she wanted to get the anesthetist to help calm her down; feelings and emotions that do not coincide with the expectations of nurses and other professional workers are often treated as symptoms and sedatives or anesthesias are used as a way of hiding these expressions from obervers who feel uncomfortable when they are expressed. The nurse also felt that she should "scold" the patient or "ignore" her, viewing these antics as "attention getting." It is useful to study the behavior of patients in relation to one's own actions toward them and expectations of them. The patient described is attempting to cover up feelings of powerlessness that may be perceived as overwhelming; she attempts to feel stronger by swearing, by giving orders to her father-in-law, and at the same time she leaves the entire process of delivering her child in the hands of strangers whom she has not known as persons who could be counted on for valuable assistance. She is so lacking in skill in this situation that her dependence upon others can be expressed only in the way she is expressing it.

When a patient says she feels inadequate, she is posing a problem that the nurse and patient can work on together. Sally, a patient who has an extensive bilateral tuberculosis is one who now has lots of time to work through her feelings about illness. When Sally was well she was inclined toward sports and other outdoor activities. Now, she becomes downhearted and asks her physician, "Will I be able to swim and to play tennis next year?" The nurse or doctor, whomever the problem is presented to, could say quite forthrightly, "Yes" or "No," whichever answer seems to apply in view of the medical evidence. But these answers do not help the patient to expand her impression of tuberculosis and what it is likely to mean in all of her future life.

What can a nurse do with Sally? A nurse might remind her that many "healthy" people are so busy they can't find time to go swimming; or that the nurse has difficulty in finding a partner and therefore has given up playing tennis. These assertions contribute nothing to an illumination of Sally's problem: "Will I play tennis or swim next year?" A nurse might interest the patient in more precise grooming of her nails, or hair, or lipstick; she might suggest books to read, letters to write, or goldfish or canaries to take care of. The patient might even comply and take on these goals of the nurse and act in accordance with them. Such busywork contributes nothing to clarification of Sally's problem as she has stated it. These suggestions cut off further communication about the problem and close the doors on Sally's attempt to validate her present experience and her future hopes with a nurse.

Symonds points out that the core of human learning is the achievement of satisfaction or avoidance of personal harm.[10, 11] Developing skill in recognizing cues in a situation and responding to those that satisfy and avoiding those that harm can occur during illness. When a nurse responds to

[10] Percival Symonds, *The Dynamics of Human Adjustment* (New York, Appleton-Century-Crofts, Inc., 1946), p. 133.
[11] See also Fig. 4, p. 34.

Sally, as a mother might to a child's curiosity about sex, saying, "You don't need to know about that today, let's feed the goldfish," the patient is forced to undergo her experience with illness in terms of genetically older experiences even though she may be striving for a more mature understanding of her problem.

A nurse might say, "You want to be able to play tennis and swim next year; let's see what is involved in that possibility." The patient might communicate her feelings about her illness as an interference to her wish to be well. When the patient has explored this as far as she wishes to go the nurse might say, "Could we take a look at what is possible now in this situation?" A helping relationship between nurse and patient is predicted on the assumption that the nurse has had greater skill and education and can therefore aid the patient to a more useful understanding of each difficulty in life that presents itself as illness of any kind is experienced.

There are many opportunities in nursing for aiding patients to become aware of their difficulties in living and for developing participant skills that are needed for solving problems that will recur in the future. When community and institutional services are co-ordinated it may become even more possible to aid citizens to prepare themselves to meet crises that arise concerning health. Each nurse can do what is possible for her in the situation in which she works. Each nurse can exercise responsibility in some degree in aiding patients to actualize their capacities when full self-realization has not occurred in previous experiences.

Summary

Illness provides an opportunity for nurses to study degrees of skill that have been developed in earlier experiences patients have had. Participation is possible when a constellation of abilities or skills—competition, compromise, co-operation, consensual validation, and love—have been developed in the process of growing up between the ages of six and fourteen.

Nurses can aid patients to identify difficulties in relation to a personal problem or one met when sharing a ward with a group of patients. Identification and discussion of the difficulty leads to expansion of the patient's first impression of a difficulty and to understanding of what are the factors or evidence on which courses of action can be based. Courses of action can be tried out and revised after further discussion with all persons affected in the situation. When nurses aid patients to face their difficulties as they arise, and in a way that aids patients to take responsibility for reaching some understanding of what is involved, goals that are set are more likely to be achieved. The patient learns skills that will be useful in later life rather than solutions to problems that may not be valid in the future. Skill in participating in the identification of a medical problem, and in designing a plan of action that leads toward a solution, is learned by the patient. Nurses can be guided by the assumption that given sufficient time, an opportunity to express oneself freely and to think through what is happening, most patients, if not all, will arrive at decisions that are best for them. The focus in the relationship of nurse to patient is on the problem. When the patient is given a chance to put the problem in his own words and to examine how he feels about it, his attitudes toward it will emerge so that he has an opportunity to examine them. Participation is required by a democratic society. When it has not been learned in earlier experiences nurses have an opportunity to facilitate learning in the present and thus to aid in the promotion of a democratic society.

Part IV. METHODS FOR STUDYING NURSING AS AN INTERPERSONAL PROCESS

Purpose: *A partial theory for the practice of nursing as an interpersonal process has been suggested in the foregoing chapters. The purpose of this section is to identify some of the opportunities that nurses have readily available and ways they can make use of them in studying what happens when a nurse and patient come together to work on a health problem. Discussion is centered on methods that a graduate nurse or students in a school of nursing can use in testing principles that have previously been outlined in this work and for expanding a theory of nursing by studying what is required of nurses by patients and communities. Further development of ways in which nursing can function as a therapeutic, educative, maturing force in society, in collaboration with workers from all other health service professions, will come from nurses who use methods that aid in explanation of what is observed in nursing situations. Clinical nursing science can contribute original insights concerning what happens among human beings who seek help when undergoing stress.*

CHAPTER 12

Observation, Communication, and Recording

Overview

OBSERVATION, communication, and recording are three interlocking operations in the nursing process. They are of utmost importance to the outcome of illness for patients and to the further development of the nurse as a person who is professionally interested in improvement in services available to people. In this chapter we are concerned in identifying principles that guide these operations and promise fuller development of clinical nursing science as a force that is useful to a dynamic, changing society. Each nurse can translate principles into action in situations in which she practices.

Observation

The aim in observation in nursing, when it is viewed as an interpersonal process, is the identification, clarification, and verification of impressions about the interactive drama, of the pushes and pulls in the relationship between nurse and patient, as they occur.[1] This impression is at first intuitively

[1] There are, of course, other functions of observation in nursing. We are concerned here with interpersonal phenomena. Students may wish to consult: Bertha Harmer and Virginia Henderson, *Textbook of the Principles and Practice of Nursing* (New York, The Macmillan Company, 1939) (4th ed.) Ch. 1. Observation of the patient.

conceived, it is a *hunch* or a generalization about what is happening in an experience. It grows out of the nurse's previous experiences in life and represents a combination of her feelings, ideas, and other evidences that have heretofore come to her attention. That is, *out of her own past experience and in the present situation each nurse will be able to express what she feels is transpiring. This hunch then becomes an hypothesis to be studied in various ways.*

The purpose in making generalizations from experiences with patients is the development of skill in the nurse in being sensitive to the problems of patients. Each nurse needs to develop such skill and to experience security and satisfaction in knowing that she can learn something valuable from each new relationship by using her own perceptions.

First impressions, or hunches, become hypotheses to be studied and therefore they affect the design of data to be gathered and analyzed at a later date. They also are generalizations to be verified or given up in future experiences with people; they may also be compared with principles stated in literature published by other professional workers. Generalizations may be tentatively verified in a group of nursing students who might validate or contradict the hunch of a particular student. In the process of talking over various hunches that have grown out of experiences of a group of student nurses, attitudes and feelings are revealed and often modified.

Hunches are largely on the sensory, subjective level at first. A nurse feels that a patient does not like women nurses, but is able to accept men nurses. This is a hunch about a particular patient. A nurse may hypothesize that a particular patient is upset when it is his turn to be taken to the operating room. In relations with several patients, she may discover that most patients are upset about forthcoming surgery. Or, she may note that patients prepared by a particular nurse are less upset than those prepared by two other nurses on a surgical section. These are all generalizations that may or may not be correct observations on what is happening in a situation.

Acting on the hypothesis that patients prepared by a particular nurse are less upset about going to the operating room, she may observe what that nurse does and come out with a hunch on how one nurse aids patients to harness energy derived from their anxiety in constructive ways; observing the other two nurses she may generalize about their lacks in preparing the patient psychologically for an operation. She may then be aided to study subsequent situations using her hypotheses about what aids patients to undergo an operation in relative comfort and what does not. Her *data will be gathered with reference to the hypotheses stated and when analyzed the findings enrich intuitive views developed in other, later situations; thus, the process develops foresight.*

In any situation the observer proceeds from impression to analysis to elaboration of the first whole impression and differentiation of related details. The first impression is an abstraction of a whole event; it is a symbol operation; it requires that a nurse can quickly take in many minute details without specifically noting any of them as she gains a broad view of what is occurring.

For example, a first impression of Fig. 11, page 220, might be that the figure represented in all of the drawings is that of "being cut off" in various ways. Closer inspection of details reveals that one drawing of the individual shows that speech is cut off and this is signified by the tied up mouth. Another shows a leg cut off; still another shows a leg partially cut off. These details when considered in relation to the first impression seem to verify the hunch identified above which can further be verified in relations with the patient as well as in case history material. Concern for the details first, before an intuitive impression has been gained, does not usually lead to a generalization but rather to rationalization of what is seen and secondary elaboration of the meaning to the observer instead of to the observed.

The difference is analogous to that between representational art, or photographic likenesses of a thing, and expressional art, which indicates the forces or pushes and pulls perceived by the artist as he sees an object or an event. Unfortunately, most readers will have had art experiences in schools where they have been asked to draw an apple, or a tulip, or a vase exactly as it is seen—that is, they are asked to gain a photographic likeness of the thing observed. Repeated experiences of this sort make it difficult to look for forces rather than things, to look for whole impressions rather than details, in experiences and events. It makes it difficult for nurses to develop sensitive hunches that can be refined with further experiences when they are immediately and overly concerned with minute details in an ongoing event.

Another example can be cited. A student reported to a college infirmary one Sunday morning and said to the nurse in charge, "I don't feel well." The nurse responded immediately, intuitively, "You look sick to me, too." This was not a routine response but an intuitive appraisal of the present situation. The nurse checked the student's temperature, pulse, and respiration and found them to be well within the range of normal. On questioning, the student offered no complaints except that she had a slight ache in the back of her head. Her color was normal, she had slept well, she had eaten a good breakfast, and in every way seemed to negate her own hunch and that of the nurse that she was sick. The nurse suggested that she stay in the infirmary for further observation. The student felt that this was an imposition on the services available, since nothing verified her feelings but she asserted, "You have more experience than I, and if you think I should stay I will." The nurse replied, "Let's put you to bed here and inquire into our hunch that you might be sick." The college physician examined the student soon afterward and on the following morning again noting that all evidence negated the hunch that the student was ill. On the third morning the student had signs of poliomyelitis, a disease that cannot be diagnosed easily in advance of symptoms of paralysis.

Nurses cannot always respond in this manner to all of their hunches but they can structure future observations in terms of them and thus increase their skill in gaining first impressions that are more nearly correct and useful.

The step in observation just outlined is in contrast to most traditional methods of observation and of teaching. In some quarters it is thought that an individual learns minute details and then puts them together into a meaningful whole. Many

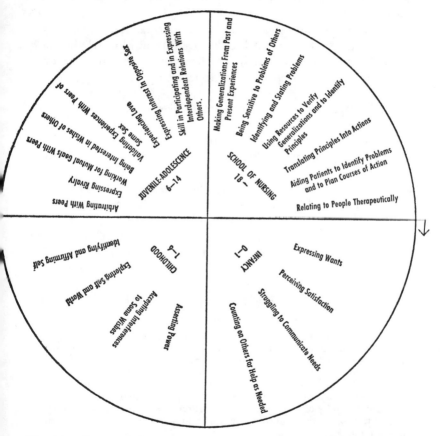

Fig. 14. Sequential arrangement of maturation of skills required for competent professional nursing.

students of the process of learning are in agreement that the reverse is true; reflecting back on information given with relation to the formation of personality it will be recalled that the infant has a first whole impression of the world and all that is contained in it; he and his mother and her breast are all one and that, to him, is all the world that is necessary. Slowly, each infant differentiates his world further and each new experience is, in turn, differentiated still further. The same concept applies in observation in interpersonal relations in nursing.

In order to study successive interpersonal relationships the student nurse refines and enlarges on her knowledge as a basis for improving skill in observation. According to Frye, a concept of good observation depends upon:[2, 3]

1. Recognition that experience carries authority of its own.
2. The scope and depth of prior knowledge the observer brings to the situations and processes studied.
3. A purpose that is clearly visualized in terms of steps to be taken.
4. An hypothesis concerning the processes or events to be studied, which the observer states in advance.
5. Adherence to the following principles:
   a) Observation is accurate when the observer notes only what is observable in a situation.
   b) Observation is complete when the requirements of the stated purpose are met.
   c) Observation is orderly when relations between parts of the data gathered can readily be seen.

[2] Adapted from: Albert M. Frye and Albert W. Levi, *Rational Belief* (New York, Harcourt, Brace & Company, Inc., 1941), pp. 342-43. A very useful text that can be consulted with profit by students in nursing.

[3] The Western Illinois State College Bulletin, *Observation in the Laboratory Schools, Macomb, Illinois,* printed by Authority of the State of Illinois, by Western Illinois State College, Vol. 28, No. 3 (January, 1949), p. 37. An excellent summary of principles of observation as they refer to teacher-education institutions; would provide a useful framework for adaptation to patient education and observation.

The most common kind of observation used in nursing is that of simply writing down whatever happens to be noted in the course of a relationship with a patient. Data obtained in this way is not precise enough for further study of it by other workers, nor does it often yield learning in terms of the purpose stated, namely, developing skill in being sensitive to problems of patients and learning something valuable from each new relationship. Lundberg refers to this kind of observation as the simplest, or *"random observation,"* in which the observer depends upon chance for data that may or may not be useful.[4] Its chief value is that of providing hypotheses for later investigation.

From initial observation, then, a nurse can determine hypotheses to be tested in the light of continuing observation of the patient. These hypotheses may have to do with the satisfaction of needs; for example, a nurse may wish to find out for herself whether it is true or not that: *when needs are met more mature needs emerge.* Her observations are then organized to find out what are the needs of the patient, how do I perform in attempting to meet them, what happens as a result; do more mature needs actually emerge? Her relations with the patient are purposeful in terms of examining hunches that she has had and giving them up when her impressions are incorrect on the basis of evidence that has been gathered.

For example, one nurse on a particular service might be designated as study-maker for particular hours during several days. Her task, then, is to sit in a strategic spot, perhaps in a medical ward, and to record the kinds of needs that are expressed by different patients and the various responses that staff make in relation to them. This data can then be analyzed in terms of the questions: What needs were emergent? How were they met? Did more mature needs follow when emergent needs were adequately met? The study-maker is

[4] George A. Lundberg, *Social Research* (New York, Longmans Green & Company, Inc., 1942), p. 6.

external to what is going on and can focus exclusively on the task of recording what is going on.

The usefulness of observation based on hypotheses, however simple, but drawn from initial impressions of the patient is in contrast to the following descriptive level reporting:[5] "A woman admitted to the ward who is about two months pregnant. Her chief complaint is that she can't eat and keep anything on her stomach and she feels so weak. She vomits even water, etc."

In order to go beyond random observation, taking a look at the patient, and writing down something on the chart as the nurse's notes for the day, it is necessary for the student nurse to employ methods that assist her in organizing her observations so that data will yield something useful and important for the welfare of the patient, and for helping her to become a keen participant-observer in nursing situations. Moreover, when nursing is viewed as an interpersonal process, a nurse cannot figuratively put the patient in a corner, write down what curious things he does, and consider that to be total observation. *In an interpersonal process it is necessary for her to view the patient as a person responding in the situation and in relation to whatever or whoever is in it with him —illusory or real.*

Observation of interpersonal relations, which are exceedingly complex at any given moment, can be facilitated by designating units of experience to be observed at any given time.[6] According to Lundberg four principles govern the arbitrary construction of units for more precise observation. (1) A unit is *appropriate* when it is useful in terms of the purpose it serves. (2) A unit is *clear* when its meaning is commonly agreed upon by all concerned in the study. (3) A unit is *measurable* when responses can be categorized in a reliable and objective way. (4) A unit is satisfactory when identified

[5] For a full discussion on the nature of hypotheses see: Frye, *op. cit.,* pp. 373-78. See also Lundberg, *op. cit.,* pp. 9-10.

[6] Lundberg, *op. cit.,* pp. 49-50.

facts can be *compared* with other data at a later period in time.

Various observers in social sciences and in psychiatry are devising useful "constructs" or units for purposes of observation that yield valuable data. For example, Baldwin, *et al.*, use the following variables to classify the behavior of parents:[7] the degree of democracy in the home, the degree of acceptance of the child; the degree of indulgence. Homes are classified as acceptant, rejectant, casual; as democratic, autocratic, and mixed; as indulgent, nonchalant, and mixed. These terms are defined in the monograph.

Lasswell points out that the context of interpersonal relations is always in terms of a variation of degrees of indulgence or deprivation.[8] These variables, indulgence and deprivation, are then further defined in terms of "activity" and "environment" making it possible for the observer to identify expectations that arise in a situation. Slavson has stated units for study of movement in relationships. These include "dominance submission," "parasitic relationships," "symbiotic," "anaclitic," "supportive," and the like.[9]

Units for study that might be useful in nursing are praise, blame, indifference, and learning. A study-maker could be assigned to gather data concerning the interpersonal relations in a particular ward with reference to the kinds of comments that patients make and the ways in which nurses use praise, blame, or indifference in relation to those comments, as well as the ways in which nurses actually aid patients to focus on learning in relation to living within the ward context.

Lasswell would make observation more precise by clarifying four key concepts in interpersonal relations:[10] "Personal-

[7] Alfred L. Baldwin, Joan Kalhorn, and Fay Huffman Bresse, *Patterns of Parent Behavior*, Psychological Monographs, Vol. 58, No. 3 (Evanston, Illinois, American Psychological Association, Northwestern University).

[8] Patrick Mullahy, *A Study of Interpersonal Relations* (New York, Hermitage House, Inc., 1949), pp. 309-63.

[9] S. R. Slavson, "Types of Relationship and Their Application to Psychotherapy," *American Journal of Orthopsychiatry*, Vol. XV, No. 2 (April, 1945), pp. 267-77.

[10] Mullahy, *op. cit.*, pp. 309-63.

ity" is the term used to refer to the way a person acts toward other persons. "Culture" is the term used to refer to the way the members of a group act in relation to one another and to other groups. A "group" is composed of persons. A "person" is an individual capable of identifying himself with others. Thus an individual is distinguished from a person; an aggregate of individuals is distinguishable from a group of persons, and the like. These concepts being clearly defined for all observers in the field make possible a variety of kinds of observation, longitudinal studies of particular variables or units for observation, cross-sectional studies of all activities concentrated over shorter periods of time, and the like.[11, 12]

Nurses have an opportunity in institutional practice to observe patients in relation to themselves and to changing events in the situation. The borders in the situation are often circumscribed and often it is possible, particularly for private duty nurses, to relate closely to the subject in the day-to-day course of events. Nursing has never tapped this valuable source for comprehensive study of interaction between nurse and patient. Private duty nurses who are able to take on the role of research worker and at the same time are able to conceive of themselves as an instrument and an object of observation in relations with patients can make an extraordinarily useful contribution to understanding of interpersonal relations in nursing. A casebook showing day-to-day accounts of what transpires between nurse and patient and its effects upon the growth of a patient is likely to come from a private duty nurse who can fit herself into the role of study-maker. Nurses also have an opportunity to study patients in relation to overlapping situations, as well as in response to strangers when crises are emergent in the life of the patient.

On admission to the hospital the patient may be said to be partaking in overlapping situations, of which the home and the new psychological situation in the hospital are representa-

---

[11] *Ibid.*, p. 324.
[12] See also: John Dollard, *Criteria for the Life History* (New Haven, Yale University Press, 1938), p. 8.

tive. As has been pointed out in Chapter 2, the patient moves from being in the home situation, becomes more fully immersed in the situation in the hospital, and gradually moves through another overlapping situation, that of the hospital and the projected or anticipated return to the situation at home.

Barker, *et al.*, have attempted to clarify the properties of the new psychological situation and the overlapping nature of other situations.[13] These hypotheses can be studied in nursing situations by nurses.

The selection of the type of "observer-observed relationship" to be used, as well as the precise units of behavior to be studied, has an important bearing on the development of observational skills in the nurse. Lasswell clarifies four types of relationships between an observer and those observed.[14] See Fig. 15, page 275. Applied to nursing, these types are: (1) The *spectator* relationship in which the patient is not aware of being observed and the nurse is outside the patient's focus of attention; for example, a nurse may be attending to the needs of one patient in a ward and at the same time observing what another patient is doing without that patient knowing it and without the nurse's attitudes or behavior entering into the situation being studied. The nurse may be observing relations between two patients in a ward while taking care of a third patient and without the first two recognizing that they are under observation. (2) The *interviewer* relationship is frequently used by nurses in clinics, in homes, when admitting patients to a hospital, and the like. The patient is more or less aware that he is being studied in some degree, that the nurse is taking note of what he is saying in response to the situation or to questions that are asked of him. The

[13] Roger Barker, Beatrice A. Wright and Mollie R. Gonick, *Adjustment to Physical Handicap and Illness: A Survey of the Social Psychology of Physique and Disability*, Bulletin 55, 1946 (230 Park Avenue, New York, Social Science Research Council).
[14] Mullahy, *op. cit.*, p. 338. See also Harold D. Lasswell, "Intensive and Extensive Methods of Observing the Personality-Culture Manifold," *Yenching Journal of Social Studies* (1938), 1:74-76.

nurse may use a prepared admission form for gathering data or she may permit the patient to take the lead in yielding data about himself and his feelings in the new situation; when the patient recognizes that he is being studied the relationship may be thought of as an interview, according to Lasswell. (3) A supervisor or director of nursing service often makes use of a *collector* relationship; that is, they make use of records or reports prepared by other nurses about patients in order to learn what has happened in a particular situation. Staff nurses and students make use of case history material gathered by internes, specialists, or other professional workers including other nurses. Partial impressions about patients are gathered through using these data from other than personal observation. (4) In *participant* relationships the nurse engages in ordinary activities connected with nursing a patient and at the same time observes the relationship between the patient and herself. The patient may refer to interest in various kinds of events, books, plays, songs, and thus give the observer cues that cannot be observed directly. The patient is aware that he is receiving nursing, such as in the form of a bath, an enema, catheterization, but he is not aware that his responses to the procedure and to the attitudes of the nurse giving it are being observed directly. The nurse as observer tries not to let the patient know that she is collecting data and that the relationship is being studied by her. Much of the data gathered is meaningful when recorded in terms of what the nurse has said and what the patient's responses to her remarks or her activities have been.

Observers may use various aids for recording data. Wire recorders or other mechanical means may be used to obtain a complete typescript, later, when the data from the relationship is transcribed for further study.[15] One nurse may act as an observer and recorder for another nurse. For example, a group of nurses were asked to spend one hour with several

[15] See: Frederick C. Redlich, John Dollard and Richard Newman, "High Fidelity Recordings of Psychotherapeutic Interviews," *American Journal of Psychiatry* (July, 1950), 107:42-48.

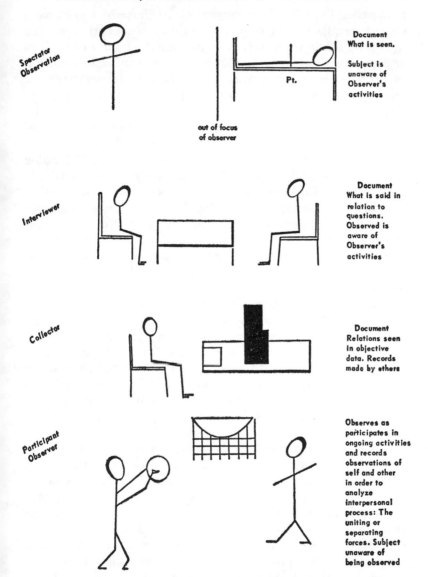

Fig. 15.   Pictorial presentation of kinds of observers, according to Lasswell.

patients taking with them large wads of clay which they were to make available to patients; two other nurses accompanied the group to the ward to remain outside the focus of activities and to record all that was observed. Television and motion pictures of patient or of nurse and patient activities may soon serve to make available important data for studying relationships of nurses and patients.

One of the main problems in the observation and study of human behavior and interaction in relations between nurses and patients is the multiplicity of factors to be studied. Some form of organization that will limit the study of unwieldy data to that which can be studied is as necessary in nursing as in any other science that studies human behavior. Lasswell suggests useful observational standpoints.[16] Nurses can organize standpoints from which they can observe what happens in a relationship with a patient. As has been cited earlier, hunches about the meaning of interaction between patients, or between the nurse and patient, can be used to guide further study. Nurses can organize observational standpoints such as *orientation* to a new situation; what is studied during the entire stay in the hospital is the way in which a patient attempts to orient himself to the new situation and to daily changes in it. What is documented includes what the patient asks for, what he questions, ways in which he uses information that is given on request or without being requested by him, what the nurse says and does in response to the patient's orienting attempts.

Nurses can organize their observations in terms of *identification, exploitation,* or *resolution* as these phases have been outlined in Chapter 2. Hypotheses suggested can be explored further or new ones can be set up on the basis of random observation of a series of patients prior to studying particular patients in an organized way. These data and the experience of collecting them will yield two products: (1) the nurse will deepen her skill in observation and become more of a scientific worker than is possible when random observation is the only method used. (2) Careful study of the nursing situation and what transpires in it will give clues to students and graduates on the kinds of demands that patients actually make, in terms of responses to their needs, and it will provide evidence on which future courses of action can be based.

Student nurses can be assisted to organize the observational standpoints and units for study as a way of making observations more precise, in the interest of developing skill and ability and of expanding their concept of nursing and what it implies. These would *move from simple units* having simple hypotheses, under which observation would take place, *to more complex interpersonal phenomena.* For example, the following organization of experiences for students might be tried out in the order suggested:

1. Simple random observation to aid the nurse in developing hunches about what transpires in her relations with one patient.
2. Spectator observations of situational frustrations in a particular ward situation.
3. Relations with a particular patient and interactions noted, in terms of ways in which the nurse interpreted and met the needs expressed.
4. Patterns of dominance or submission used individually in group meetings of a class of students in the school.
5. Observing in a group of students, or in a relationship with a patient, for responses that serve to unite the group or the nurse and patient.
6. Observing in a group of students, or in a relationship with a patient, for responses that seem to separate the group or the nurse and patient.
7. Random observation for hunches about internal frustrations and expressions of anxiety, and transformation of its energy into a pattern of behavior, in a relationship with a patient. State hypotheses to be studied.
8. Study hypotheses stated for a brief period in order to get hunches about courses of action a nurse might take in

relations with that patient, in order to aid the patient to grow and to develop more productive relations with others.

9. Admission of a series of patients to study factors in the new psychological experience, from the standpoint of pushes and pulls toward overlapping situations and the directional bearing of the patient's responses to the nurse and family members.

10. Study of orientation needs of patients in relations with nurses.

11. Observation of the movement of relationship patterns in a long term relationship with reference to psychological tasks and learning, with a patient in a hospital or home.

12. Multilateral relations in a ward environment, including frustration, anxiety, and conflict and their effects or interaction with one nurse and a group of patients.

13. Use of Form #1, see Fig. 17, p. 308, with counseling by an instructor or other professional person competent to give the help required, as a way of studying unique and recurring patterns in the relations of nurse to patient with a problem centering around or including the oral zone, *i.e.*, a tonsillectomy, a thyroidectomy, dental work, or jaw fracture.

14. Use of Form #1 and counseling, as a way of studying relations with a patient admitted for treatment concerning the gastrointestinal tract, *i.e.*, peptic ulcer, colostomy, appendectomy, and the like.

15. Use of Form #1 and counseling, as a way of studying relations with a patient facing an anal problem, *i.e.*, a hemorrhoidectomy, anal pruritus, rectal fissure, etc.

16. Use of Form #1 and counseling, as a way of studying relations with a patient admitted for treatment of the genital tract, *i.e.*, a circumcision, gynecological treatment or surgery.

17. Use of Form #1 with counseling, as a way of studying relations with a patient whose problem involves manipulation or destruction of bodily areas useful for creative

functions, *i.e.*, pregnancy and delivery, at term or miscarriage, amputation of an arm for an individual who needs that arm in his productive work, etc.

18. Use of Form #1 and counseling, as a way of studying relations with a patient whose problems center around an organ of sensation or perception, as an eye, ear, nose, throat.

Other sequences of observational experiences might be designed for the specific needs of particular nurses or nurse groups. Each would involve, preferably, a study of the unique and recurring patterns in relations of nurses and patients, generalizations from personal experience followed by study of case material and the literature. This kind of study provides educational opportunities for student and graduate nurses to develop sensitivity to the problems of patients studied, and it provides leads for the development of courses of action that a nurse might follow when the evidence on which these can be based has been accumulated and understood. It provides a focus for study and for identifying and correlating previous insights and knowledge with relation to problems the nurse faces every day with patients; it develops a method for study that leads to the collection of evidence as a basis for designing experiences for patients that will aid them to use illness for learning and improving skills needed to cope with problems in future experiences.

Role-playing is a way of improving skill in observation.[17] It serves to aid observers and the observed to identify what is happening in a situation in which both participate. For example, a group of nurses were studying the problem: What are the feelings involved in being rejected? A smaller group within the large class role-played a discussion about a film during which everything that one student said was accepted and everything that another student said was rejected. These two students were not told, in advance, that the other four

[17] P. M. Symonds, "Role Playing as a Diagnostic Procedure in the Selection of Leaders," *Sociatry* (1947), 1:43-52.

students in the smaller group were planning to relate to them in these ways. Rejection and acceptance were role-played as a way of aiding the four students to become aware of ways in which they viewed these two forms of behavior in their relations with others and as a way of aiding two of the students to experience and to relate to the class how they felt about what happened during the experience.

A nurse might role-play with a patient the way in which he will go through a procedure, such as a basal metabolism, or the way in which he might undergo a job interview after rehabilitation from a long illness. Role-playing may be designed or accidental; patients often demonstrate verbally or with gestures how another patient or individual has acted; nurses often re-enact for their roommates a scene that took place in the office of the instructor or the director. These are ways of reliving an experience in order to expand its meaning in awareness or they may be ways of undergoing future experiences in order to develop the necessary insights and skills in relations to feelings about future events. They also serve to provide observational data about individual responses and interactions between persons.

When the nurse observes in ward situations she recognizes the same tensions, transformations of energy, and processes of interpersonal relations at work that are seen in individual situations with one patient. Likewise, she recognizes that there are functions that go on in the group itself whether the nurse is present or not. These functions include that of leadership. Leadership functions are carried or assigned to individuals who keep the group process moving. A group of patients engaged in discussion, when observed, will show that one patient serves as leader or that this function is passed around as the discussion turns from one problem to another. Often this is not an organized aspect of the work of the group; that is, the patients do not stop and decide who will be their leader. But, certain patients tend to keep the group focused on the issue under discussion; when there is a proclivity to wander each individual tells some different experience. Or, one patient may aid in identifying an individual in the group who can function as a resource person; a nurse might be called in to answer a specific question that the group has, such as: "Nurse, is the doctor going to make rounds today or isn't he?"

Various functions of members of a group may be observed. One patient may serve to support patients who need ego support, another may be hypercritical of the hospital and of individuals present, another may function as arbitrator between two patients who view a problem differently and who seem unable to struggle for common agreement. Nurses can study what happens in groups of patients that aids the processes of self-repair and that is not ordinarily available through the nurses' relations with patients. It is conceivable that a patient who is physically helpless and dependent upon the nurse also needs at some time to be in a situation that approximates what transpires during the course of development of personality between the ages of six and sixteen; that is, it is more difficult to aid a patient to grow when confined to a private room during a long and sustained illness in which dependent relations are an outstanding feature without providing an opportunity for the patient to mix with others at a point in the course of illness. The possibility is analogous to that of a child whose overprotective mother does not permit him to have a group of friends and later a chum, and whose only contacts with children occur in a formal school where communication is largely restricted to that which occurs between teacher and each pupil. Since the hypothesis suggested above has not been studied in nursing, evidence as to its validity is not available for designing nursing in a way most useful for patients.

Groups of patients may be studied from the standpoint of the psychological tasks that are being re-enacted and the degrees of skill that patients use in the direction of participation in the work of a patient group, as defined by them. They may be observed from the standpoint of the *cohesion* that occurs and the basis for it; other observational standpoints might be *interest level,* degrees of *member acceptance* of each other (sometimes measured by the use of a sociogram), by the degrees of reliance upon authoritative direction from nurses and others.

Groups of patients may be observed from the standpoint of *interfering* or disjunctive forces involved. These may have to do with mechanical difficulties, as in the physical facilities that are available and restrict activities, failure to arbitrate or to view differences, failure to communicate or assenting by default with what one more verbal member asserts is the difficulty in a particular ward. They have to do with *negative compelling forces* in the interpersonal relations, such as internal frustrations, conflict, anxiety, tensions, individual prestige needs, personifications that operate outside awareness, and the like. *Positive compelling forces* include listening attentively and expanding what has been said in light of one's own experience in contrast to swallowing it or introducing a new and different idea. Clarifying the feelings of others, seeking clarification in what has been said, working for understanding of the problem under discussion—these are ways of improving a situation. Another way of severing relations in groups is the development of cliques within the ward group, or *scapegoat* assignments to one patient who becomes the butt of the other patients' jokes or derogatory remarks; these serve to split patients into smaller groups and thus to destroy what may be therapeutic functions of the whole group in a ward situation.

While the nurse is often a participant member in group activities and interests that make up the life in any hospital ward, student nurses should have supervised experiences before they are asked to take on full responsibility. Observation of groups and recording these observations for study of the dynamics at interplay among members can occur in the groups of students who work in various wards or who are seeking to understand a particular problem that nurses face. Studying the process of relations with other students is an important element in the study of interpersonal relations in nursing since the nurse needs to be able to recognize how she relates to individual patients as well as to groups of nurses in her preprofessional associations with them.[18] Knowledge of group dynamics and practice in observing what occurs assists the student to assume the role of change-agent in any group of patients, a role in which patients often cast her when they spontaneously re-experience older feelings of rivalry with siblings or with peers. These earlier difficulties are frequently relived in wards as patients undergo illness as an experience; a nurse can aid in making current human relations significant in terms of growth.

When patients cluster around one or two nurses, symbolic of mothers or of women figures in the culture, the nurse often is placed in the position of functioning as an arbitrator of feelings and attitudes. Transforming these experiences into events that are educative requires an understanding of the dynamics of relationships in groups of two or more persons.

The nurse is a participant observer in most relationships in nursing. This requires that she use herself as an instrument and as an object of observation at the same time that she is participating in the interaction between herself and a patient or a group. The more precise the nurse can become in the use of herself as an instrument for observation, the more she will be able to observe in relation to performances in the nursing process. The analysis of interaction between nurse and patient yields data as a basis for improving nursing practice. All nursing judgments in practice grow out of participant-observation. While professional purposes, ethical ideals, technological hypotheses, and a diagnosis of the patient's disease are all held to be important to the development of sound nursing practice, *nurses—like other human beings—act on the basis of the meaning of events to them, that is, on the basis of their immediate interpretation of the climate and the performances that transpire in a particular*

---

[18] For a list of processes studied by psychoanalysts see: H. S. Sullivan, *Conceptions of Modern Psychiatry* (Washington, D.C., William Alanson White Psychiatric Foundation, 1947), pp. 46-48.

relationship. At the same time, the patient will act on the basis of the meaning of his illness to him. *The interaction of nurse and patient is fruitful when a method of communication that identifies and uses common meanings is at work in the situation.*[19]

The recognition of this basic principle leads to the conclusion that specific forms of conduct cannot be demanded or assured by administration, supervision, and by instructional staff except to the degree that individuals who represent these authorities responsible for service provide opportunity for nurses to examine the meaning of events to them, so that such meaning can operate in awareness. An administrator or supervisor may consistently demonstrate behavior that they wish emulated by others in the situation. But, the quality of expression in the rendering of nursing service is an outcome of what is observed, and of more or less spontaneous and considered behavior occurring in response to unenforceable laws, promptings arising within each nurse that are internal, basic, and personal. When these promptings can be examined openly, as an aspect of basic education, or as a component of in-service education, they become more and more amenable to control as they are more fully understood and often can be brought in line with purposes and ideals that are common to all who function within a particular service. Each nurse can learn to observe that the rewards in nursing are qualities that nurses impart to others during illness or during professional relations; in the same vein, slipshod, needful, vindictive personal relationships, however portrayed, are basic modes of responding that are demanded by the self of the individual as a selective organizer and responder to experience.

Observation precedes interpretation of the collected facts. Adaptation to or learning in a situation precedes its integration, as a life experience. Both observation and interpretation depend upon seemingly isolated impressions of a sensory

[19] See also communication, p. 289.

or bodily nature and out of a mound of data there occurs an organized conception, in some degree, a refinement of an initial impression or hunch. For the nurse, this represents her conclusive findings in a particular relationship at its termination. Meanwhile, the nurse responds in the situation and makes judgments in practice that seem relevant at the time. At the close of a relationship evaluation of findings refines knowledge that will be useful in the future, rather than to the patient with whom data has been collected. Future hypotheses can be enriched by full evaluation of each foregoing experience and serve as a way of clarifying for the nurse the meaning of events that have transpired and that may now be integrated in the stream of experiences already undergone.

Similarly, the patient arrives at a final conception of his experience with illness. It is a larger view than that held initially and if his relations with nurses have been rewarding, in terms of needs met and feelings clearly recognized in awareness, the patient can integrate the experience as one among others met in life. From a first whole impression through a multitude of detailed and related experiences at the hands of nurses and others, the self of the patient selects a view that symbolizes the total event and integrates it into the backlog of experiences previously undergone. If the integration is sound, and the patient "knows" by way of his feelings that he has experienced something meaningful to him in terms of learning, the patient can proceed to other new and informing experiences. If the integration is not sound, doubts and "felt difficulties" will continue to arise in relation to the self or security needs of the patient. For both the nurse and the patient the integrating tendencies come from the self-system and its needs for self-enhancement, prestige, clarity, and its need to avoid anxiety.

While the nurse observes in relation to an hypothesis or other units of observation, and the patient observes in relation to some vaguely conceived goal, such as health, yet, it is during observation and adaptation that *both undergo tensions and needs of a multitudinous variety.* According to Sullivan, *ultimately, all that can be observed is the way in which energy deriving from needs, tensions, and anxiety is transformed into relations with other individuals.*[20] When needs are met, tensions are relieved in productive or nonproductive ways and adaptations that work to relieve anxiety have been adopted by nurse and patient, a state of relative calm is reached in which tensions are largely abated—the issue is decided, the energy is transformed into behavior, actions have been determined.

Much depends upon whether observation and adaptation occur in automatic fashion, that is unguided by awareness, or whether purposeful direction comes from a self largely aware of movement and meaning of events in the experience in progress. Automaton behavior is revealed in repetition of earlier patterns that worked in previous situations; fruitful learning is characterized by the development in the situation of new patterns of response dependent upon the new situation and its meaning to the observer.

Activity that is guided by an ever growing awareness of the forces at work in the self in action is the only form of behavior that is useful to the nurse who would act therapeutically in relations with patients. As has been said before, while all such therapeutic relationships are contingent upon collaborative actions and responsibility shared with physicians and other professional workers, yet there is the central fact that the patient learns something from the nurse relating to him. This inescapable and observable fact demands professional consideration.

Ability to observe, to understand, and to interpret interaction are prerequisite to making ever more useful judgments in practice. A distinction may be made between judgments in

[20] H. S. Sullivan, "Tensions Interpersonal and International: A Psychiatrist's View," p. 83. Paper in Hadley Cantril (ed.), *Tensions That Cause Wars* (Urbana, University of Illinois Press, 1950).

practice and judgments in fact.[21] Consideration in this differentiation as they affect nursing, are as follows:

Judgments in practice:

1. Nurses are always in situations where something has to be done; choice is permitted by the necessity for a decision on what *should* be done.
2. While predetermined policies may operate to guide nurse conduct, choices among alternatives are often possible.
3. Choices depend upon the deliberation of facts.

Judgments in fact:

1. When facts are considered choice is further limited.
2. Facts determine what *can* be done, *i.e.,* what the possibilities and limits are.

A continuum of these two types of judgments operates in nursing. Nurses move from judgments in practice to those in fact, which, in effect, make future judgments in practice sounder and more immediately effective. Thus, in connection with certain disease entities or, for example, an amputation of a leg, whether cure is possible or not, or whether the function of the leg can be restored or not, can be judged as facts. However, in interpersonal situations, facts are not always as easily demonstrable as in the more clear-cut medical-surgical problems. Regarding "cure" of participation in life by withdrawal, or by destructive assault on others, facts that determine what can be done are difficult to narrow into discrete assertions. As nurses develop and test experiences with patients who manifest nonproductive participation in

[21] Clifford Woody (general ed.), *The Discipline of Practical Judgment in a Democratic Society,* Yearbook No. 28, of the National Society of College Teachers of Education (Chicago, Ill., University of Chicago Press), 1943. See also: S. E. Asch, "Studies in the Principles of Judgments and Attitudes: II Determination of Judgments by Group and by Ego Standards," *Journal of Social Psychology* (1940), 12:433-445.

life such as these, and as their findings are pooled with those of other professional workers, facts on which judgments can be based will become available for use.

In making judgments in practice in nursing situations, particularly with reference to relations with patients, decisions may be useful only in specific situations and may not apply to the next patient. Each individual's modes of responding are variously determined, and thus are different, making it difficult to pin down the variables for purposes of standardization of the behavior of nurses.

Policies, when determined in advance by the professional group for whom they are expected to operate, act as a formulated and general basis for action. They must always be kept open for revision following further observations. Since policies are based on experience and on decisions actually made in practice in the *past,* when subsequent use reveals exceptions to these general guides, reformulation of policies and hence reshaping of subsequent decisions occurs. Hence policies and principles that guide action are hypotheses that are held open to revision and reconstruction following observation.

For example, a group of nurses might decide that the following policy would operate in relation to the behavior of patients: *Patients have the right to be as sick as they need to be* (in terms of aggressive behavior, for instance) *in order to get well.* Then it may be found that this policy interferes with another one also set up, such as: *The welfare of a group of patients is a more important consideration than the private concerns of the individual patient.* Observation has shown that these two policies cannot operate side by side in the present situation. Reformulation of policy, in order to harmonize and to retain the useful aspects of both, might lead to this one: *Patients have the right to be as sick as they need to be in order to get well, but it is sometimes necessary to intervene and provide individual arrangements in order that the exercise of that right does not seriously interfere with the rights and progress of other patients.*

The making of judgments in practice is basic to problem-solving. Observation and understanding of what is observed are essential operations for making judgments and for designing experiences with patients that aid them in the solution of their problems.

Communication

The development of consciousness of tools used in nursing includes awareness of means of communication; spoken language, rational and nonrational expressions of wishes, needs, and desires, and the body gesture.

Nurses use words in many ways in their relations with patients. They communicate facts, they converse about everyday events, they convey interpretations of events that occur in carrying out the plan of treatment. Word consciousness in these aspects of communication tends to influence the developing relationship in the direction of improved learning for both participants.[22] Concepts, words, or symbols chosen to express ideas, thoughts, or feelings, or to indicate objects referred to, often determine whether the tool—language—will be helpful in the reshaping of experience or whether it will operate as a detriment to elaboration of meanings of events.[23] Each concept or word has both a referent and a reference.[24] The word is the symbol; the reference is its meaning held in the mind of its user; and the referent is the actions or object the symbol signified.[25]

Words are not the only symbols. A nurse can be viewed as a symbol of an earlier relationship and through her actions

---

[22] C. K. Ogden and I. A. Richards, *The Meaning of Meaning* (New York, Harcourt, Brace & Company, Inc., 1945). Word consciousness as the definition of semantics.

[23] P. W. Bridgman, *The Logic of Modern Physics* (New York, The Macmillan Company, 1927), pp. 5-7, ". . . the concept is synonymous with the corresponding set of operations."

[24] See Fig. 1, p. 5.

[25] For a useful reference on the use and meaning of symbols see: Frye, *op. cit.*

come to stand for or personify a mother or some other cultural figure in the mind of the patient.

The aim in communication is the selection of symbols or concepts that convey both the reference, or meaning in the mind of the individual, *and the referent, the object or actions symbolized* in the concept. When two individuals using the same word hold the same meaning and identify the same operations of the meaning in action, communication is fruitful. For example, two nurses using the word democracy would, if each understood the other, have approximately the same meaning in their minds and both would use the same actions in acting on the meaning of the word that was held. Since this is an achievement of considerable importance but difficult in accomplishment, *a second aim in communication can be stated as the wish to struggle toward the development of common understanding of the kind described above.*

The language used in relations between nurses and patients, that is, the words that will ensure useful communication, cannot be determined in advance. However, two principles can be used to guide the development of communication, or it may largely be determined by method, as in counseling.[26] Two main principles are:

1. *Clarity:* Words and sentences used are clarifying events when they occur within the frame of reference of common experience of both or all participants, or when their meaning is established or made understandable as a result of joint and sustained effort of all parties concerned.
2. *Continuity:* Continuity in communication occurs when language is used as a tool for the promotion of coherence or connections of ideas expressed and leads to discrimination of relationships or connections among ideas and the feelings, events, or themes conveyed in those ideas.

[26] In this connection the nondirective method of counseling is noteworthy. See: Carl Rogers, *Counseling and Psychotherapy* (Boston, Houghton Mifflin Company, 1942). Virginia Axeline, *Play Therapy* (Boston, Houghton Mifflin Company, 1947).

With respect to the principle of clarity, referring back to Chapter 1, it can be noted that the word nurse becomes clearer in the minds of a group of nurses when they talk over what is meant and when they decide together on the actions symbolized in the word nurse. In relations with patients, the meaning of nurse to the nurse and to the patient is often quite different. Each has preconceptions about the meaning of the word and about the actions that portray its meaning. A common reference for the word can be arrived at through observation and discussion, as each learns to identify the preconceptions of the other and connects the reference with the actual actions of a particular nurse. Nurses often aid patients in getting clear on earlier views of a nurse. Views not reflected in the actions of the present nurse may be held because the patient holds to an impossibly idealistic conception of a nurse. In general, a nurse can assist the patient in clarifying the relationship of earlier preconceptions by permitting expression of feelings and by sustaining a new referent that is worth while and more acceptable.

Clarity is promoted when the meaning to the patient is expressed and talked over and a new view is expanded in awareness. This is true of the concept of nurse as well as his view of the problem, feelings about himself, and the like.

Occasionally words are used that give rise to discomfort in a patient. For example, a child hospitalized for fracture of the femur heard her physician say, "You can take her upstairs this afternoon." The child became anxious and fearful and nurses were unable to identify the basis for her behavior. Finally the child revealed that she was apprehensive about returning to the operating room, which is what "upstairs" meant to her. The nurses were able to clarify what was meant, that "upstairs" this time referred to a trip to the X-ray department which happened to be in the same direction as the operating room.

Clarity also refers to an understanding of the meaning through some degree of identification of the operations or referents to which a word points. For example, in this culture, the word death often gives rise to disturbances in feelings. One group questioned about what "to die" means indicated the following references in the minds of its members: "the end," "sleep," "relief from pain," "escape," "it is painful to die," "moving from the known to the unknown," "a struggle," "going away," "separation from others," "unclutching, that is to release what one has," "the body dies," "the self or person dies." It can be seen that one of the central themes in the foregoing individual meanings seems to be that of cutting off contacts with people, letting go of people and things without opportunity for turning back again. This same group then identified the referents for the word death, namely, the feelings and behavior that indicate or show the approach of death. The usual physical signs including gasping for breath were identified. Other operations were "being detached or acting as if detached from one's surroundings," "acting resigned," "an anxious expression on the face," "quick motion of the head and eyes," "looking about and pleading for help in vain," "excitement," "antagonisms," "struggling or fighting," the complaint "I can't breathe." The central theme in these ways of behaving that signify death seems to be that of powerlessness, complete helplessness and dependence upon others in facing the emergent problem: aloneness in the face of impending death. Understanding the meaning of the word and of the experience of death, as it appears to patients, in the context given above also suggests the nursing problem: How to help this patient to engage whatever remaining rational power he has available to make the most useful last choices concerning closing his life? One aspect of the solution of this problem, on the part of nurses, may be that of making available to the patient resources offered through the clergy; another might be that of working through emergent feelings in the presence of other family members. Whatever actions a nurse deems useful are likely to grow out of her understanding of the cultural meaning of death, her own personal references for it, as well as what it means to each patient in a situation that can be understood.

Continuity is promoted when the nurse is able to pick up threads of conversation that the patient offers in the course of a conversation and over a longer period such as a week and when she aids the patient to focus and to expand these threads. Opportunities for elaboration and for connecting older meanings with present events, and for evaluating them in terms of new possibilities in the current situation, abound in nursing situations. For example, a patient may say, "I've been wanting someone to talk to all afternoon but the nurses were busy." Continuity is possible when the nurse responds in terms of, "You felt like talking to someone." If the nurse responded, "I know, I've been busy, too," the thread is taken away from the patient and the nurse's activities are posed as a possible avenue for discussion; that is, the patient is more likely to say, "You have been busy, too; what have you been doing?" This may be a way of ensuring attention from the nurse, focusing on her work, her activities. Yet, when the feelings of the patient are seen as being in need of examination and further connection with present events the nurse's injection of self into the continuity of ideas acts as an interference to exploration of the patient's feelings. It is sometimes erroneously thought to be helpful to divert a patient from thinking about himself. A nurse would have to be perceptive of the aloneness inherent in the remark, "I've been wanting to talk to someone all afternoon . . ." and know that there must be something of importance the patient wishes to discuss in order to get a clearer meaning of what is happening in the present situation.

Often the nurse may not understand the meaning of what is wanted by the patient, or of what is said. It is always possible to ask: What did you have in mind? Have I heard you correctly? Have I understood what you mean, let me repeat what you said? Perhaps you can help me to get clear on what you mean? Perhaps both of us are looking at this issue or problem from a different standpoint; maybe we'd better talk about its meaning to each. I do it this way for these reasons but perhaps you have better reasons for wanting it done some other way? These ways of framing questions, when questions are used, help the patient to reformulate what he has said and they tend to bring out into the open differences that always exist when two people relate to each other.

Picking up what the patient has said and making use of it for elaborating and expanding the relationship gives a feeling of prestige and importance to patients. It makes what has been said by them take on new meaning, for if it is important enough for the nurse to listen the patient is more likely to pay attention to what he is actually saying. He becomes more critical of his expressions and exerts more effort to clarify them.

According to Langer, "reality" is woven out of the various signs and symbols that occur during experiences in life. Experience calls our attention to cues, or signs, to which we then attend; symbolization is the process by which these cues are linked up, and connections, tranformations, and continuities of experience become the "tissue" of "reality." Each sign attended to becomes the context for the next sign.[27] It has already been pointed out in this work that learning occurs as the patient comes to attend to cues in the situation as he perceives them, rather than in response to cues or commands from others. Attending to cues is possible and is reinforced when the nurse focuses her attention on what the patient is saying and aids the patient in clarifying and in connecting ideas and feelings to the present illness and his experience with professional workers.

Language is used in communication to express conceptions, to describe experiences, to point to or signify other realities.[28] It may also be used to avoid conveying concep-

---

[27] Suzanne K. Langer, *Philosophy in a New Key* (Cambridge, Harvard University Press, 1942), p. 280.
[28] *Ibid.,* pp. 282-83.

tions or feelings, that is, to prevent communication. Or, words may be used to convey meanings that are hidden, that underlie the words used but are not conveyed directly within them. That is, "word salads" or sentences that are not immediately intelligible to the hearer may be in the mood: I dare you to find out what I am thinking or saying.

In nursing it is necessary to find out more than the patient tells directly. Indirect communication occurs through words and through actions that can be desymbolized and their hidden meaning identified or at least speculated upon. Figs. 11 and 12 (pp. 220, 227) are illustrations of indirect communications between people. The patient who cannot fall asleep unless she holds the nurse's hand at night is communicating something resembling a childlike need for protection and sheltering in the face of a crisis or an event that is not fully understood. Symptomatic acts such as vomiting, where there is no evidence of physical or organic reason for this rejection of food, are often symbolic of one who feeds, of an idea, of an experience in the past or in the future.

Nurses can ask themselves, in most situations, what the patient is saying through his complaints about his bodily functioning, about personnel, about his family. *What is the patient saying that he cannot say in any other way?* What is the language of his illness? What does it communicate indirectly about the individual who is sick? [29] In order to understand the language of the illness, to determine what the symptom says that the patient cannot express directly, it is necessary to take what is actually said by a patient, the manifest content of the communication so-to-speak, and to desymbolize and interpret it for possible hunches to the underlying meaning. This means simply that when a nurse charts, "the patient complains of headache," she has overabstracted in most cases and has denied herself and others an opportunity to analyze valuable data. This is particularly

[29] For a particularly helpful discussion see: Flanders Dunbar, *Your Child's Mind and Body* (New York, Random House, Inc., 1949), p. 188.

true if the patient says, "I have a beating pain in my head," or, "I feel as though someone was hitting me on the head with a sledge hammer." The exact words of the patient can be scrutinized in relation to other case history or day-to-day findings in the nursing situation. It may be discovered that

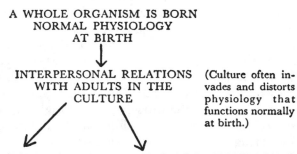

A WHOLE ORGANISM IS BORN
NORMAL PHYSIOLOGY
AT BIRTH

↓

INTERPERSONAL RELATIONS   (Culture often in-
WITH ADULTS IN THE   vades and distorts
CULTURE   physiology that
                            functions normally
                            at birth.)

MEANING OF INTERPERSONAL   MEANING OF INTERPERSONAL
EVENTS TO ADULTS   EVENTS TO GROWING CHILD

(Conflicting meanings can be clarified leading
to satisfaction or distorted to bring relief from
anxiety.)

(Is this the area in which ideas and meanings
of events begin to influence and to bring about
chemical and structural distortions in the organism?)

↓

WHOLE ORGANISM RESPONDING
(To events and perceived meaning of them.)

PARTIAL EXPERIENCES   WHOLE EXPERIENCE
IDENTIFIED   IS EXPANDED

(In order to clarify parts of a whole   (Understanding of experience leads to
experience or to experience relief from new problems and to new whole ex-
anxiety.)   periences.)

FEELINGS SYMBOLIZED
IN NONRATIONAL
EXPRESSIONS

Fig. 16.   A relationship of meaning to events
and to physiological functioning.

in the past this patient has actually been beaten, literally and figuratively, in relations with parents and peers and that now he is taking on that function himself, as indicated by a beating pain in the head. Dunbar points out that children often use organ behavior to express feelings that cannot be verbalized directly; older children and adults have picked up conventional clichés and often use these as clichés rather than as actual expressions of feeling. There is need for nurses to be able to discriminate the importance and meaning of what is said.

When the principle that the self is a selective organizer and responder in experience is kept in mind it can be seen that a nurse can say one thing and the *patient will hear according to his own selective responses.* It is on this basis that patients are often unable to be receptive to advice; in lay terms, it is said that "they hear what they want to hear." [30] More accurately, they hear selectively in terms of older experiences and the need to avoid anxiety by restricting their awareness of what is said.

The primary concern of nurses in communications with patients is the development with the patient of a clear and adequate conception of the experience with illness. Perception, thought, recall, the view of self, tendencies such as selective inattention and dissociation all operate in some degree for every patient. The patient's initial impression of illness, as an experience that is happening to him, requires sharper differentiations and meaningful expansion as the event itself undergoes changes as a direct result of relations with nurses, doctors, other professional workers, and other patients. Nursing functions to assist the patient in gaining a breadth of view in relation to this ongoing experience as the patient undergoes it so that a clear conception of its relation to his life in the future can be seen and accepted by the patient.

Words are symbols that can be used to facilitate relations between people or they may serve to disunite them further. Consciousness of the meaning and use of words requires

[30] See p. 46, p. 229.

awareness of self. Ability to recognize the meaning and the actions implied in words, or concepts, or principles, and to relate them to everyday nursing practice improves practices at the same time leading to sounder personality organization. The alternative is to have a more or less clear meaning of words and to act out on the basis of motivations and needs that derive from personality or character, outside awareness and without correspondence to the words used. Adequate conceptualization implies that the word or concept, the reference, and the corresponding operations or acts will be harmonious to a considerable degree; and that the process or steps in the total operation will be recognized in a way that leads to the development of experiences with patients that take them through the steps toward adequate conceptualization.

Nursing practice can be improved when such words as "love," "respect for the patient," and "nursing the whole patient" are clear to those nurses who find these symbols useful in communication. The operations which denote showing love, showing respect, and rendering care to "the whole patient" have not yet been adequately identified and relationships to the references in the minds of nurse practitioners clarified. What these words or phrases mean to each member of a group of ten nurses and to the ten patients with whom they are having contacts could be investigated for further evidence of the disparity that so often exists between the references and the referents for which these symbols stand.

Rational attitudes and communication are those of which the participant is aware, recognizing connections between the meaning of an idea and the actions related to it, or between the behavior expressed and the traits of character of the individual whose behavior is being studied. Nonrational attitudes and communications are governed by traits of character of which the subject is unaware; they often govern behavior that occurs automatically, without recognition of underlying relationships. Character, as Fromm has defined it, represents basic orientations to life which require certain forms of participation in life.[31]

Fromm has conceptualized a continuum of character types of which the two following categories represent polar constructs: (1) Those persons in whom security is felt as an active result of recognition of self as one who achieves something because of being related to others in worth-while endeavor. (2) Those individuals whose sense of security derives from following others, passively expressing expectations without participation in or productive relatedness to the world.

In terms of orientations to life, these two constructs point to two ideal types: (1) Those oriented to the future, looking ahead incessantly, considering the present in its perspective, and making minimum reference to the past except as it aids in interpretation of present events and future possibilities. (2) Those oriented to the past, looking back upon the past longingly, or toward death as the main reference point in the future.

It is well to bear in mind that these ideal types, or polar constructs, represent opposite ends of a continuum on which the character and attitudes of all persons are expressed in varying intensities.

Types falling under the first categories discussed are more likely to express attitudes in a rational, or consciously directed, manner. Those falling along the opposite pole of the continuum, are more likely to have many attitudes operating outside awareness, and therefore outside the reach of self-control in particular situations. Nonrational expressions, however, occur in some intensity as human events for all people, the main point to be kept in mind being that of developing nursing as a method which is valid for furthering self-recognition of one's own nonrational ways of experiencing and of relating to others.

From the standpoint of interpersonal relations, it has

[31] Erich Fromm, *Man for Himself* (New York, Rinehart & Co., Inc., 1947). This valuable contribution to the understanding of the formation of character and its relations to behavior provides many leads for nurses who want to understand themselves and their patients.

already been pointed out that a patient or a nurse may relate to "illusory figures" or personifications, anonymous authorities that operated during formative years in earlier situations and that still function to direct, guide, or govern the individual outside awareness. Parental prohibitions and standards incorporated into personality were communicated personally in earlier years; in present situations they are communicated through the self, which is made up of "reflected appraisals," which, in many instances, have not been reworked and discarded when necessary. Older appraisals can be critically re-evaluated by any individual in the light of his adult needs and the meaning of new situations; often this requires therapeutic intervention for full expansion of personality. Likewise, the growing nurse arrives at a point where she can evaluate all of her former nursing instructors and supervisors as people, recognizing their strengths and their weaknesses, rather than being forever subservient to their teachings and admonitions without further appraisal of new and recent experiences of self. The professional nurse who becomes ever more mature recognizes the contribution of the great nurses of the past without being intimidated or dominated by their contributions to the exclusion of consideration of all new possibilities in the light of a changing social situation. Many rigidities in nursing education and practice are outcomes of communication of traditional standards that have not been re-evaluated in the light of present circumstances.

Nonrational expressions are also manifested in a cultural way, in myths, dreams, rituals, folk tales, folk songs, and the like.[32] These communicate in a less clear and a less directly expressed manner many cultural, intellectual, and emotional issues that affect patients. The longings, hopes, and fears that confront people in a culture in their search for recog-

[32] J. Louise Despert, "Psychosomatic Study of Fifty Stuttering Children," *American Journal of Orthopsychiatry*, Vol. XVI, No. 1 (January, 1946), pp. 100-32. See particularly a series of fables used to test "sensitive areas" in family and emotional life. Erich Fromm, *The Forgotten Language* (New York, Rinehart & Co., Inc., 1951).

nition and understanding are expressed in disguised form.

Nonrational expressions can best be understood by recognition of the nature and purpose of the process of symbolization. Symbols such as words are uttered to indicate something for which they stand and which cannot be adequately expressed in any other way. Pictures, diagrams, markings of various sorts are also symbols that communicate meanings to others.

Words, as they are used in ordinary communication, usually carry rational meaning. That is, such words as table, chair, book, dog are understood in a general way by all participants since they fall within the common experience of most people. The meaning of words used is essentially dependent upon shared experiences and this possibility is more likely to occur when a word symbolizes concrete things rather than individual perceptions or experiences that are unique. Socialization and rationalization play a large part in the choice of words used for everyday conversation.

Language is generally used to designate objects, express thoughts in conventionally or socially recognizable ways. That is, communication about these external processes are ways of sharing an experience verbally with others. Symbolization is the process that combines the meaning of a visualized or perceived object or event and the meaning of the word or idea that stands for them. It is a means for rational communication that is both necessary and economical of time.

Symbols are also representative of emotional ideas or desires; they may be interpreted in order to reveal underlying themes, wishes or wants that cannot be expressed directly. These are referred to as nonrational expressional forms of human nature. For example, when dreams, fairy tales, or current song hits are analyzed the way is opened for understanding the emotional feelings that underlie the words and sentences used.

Although the structure of symbols is the same in myths, folk songs, fairy tales, etc., the technique for interpretation of the meaning of dreams has been more highly developed through the practice and advancement of psychoanalysis. All nonrational expressions are susceptible to interpretation through use of method more like that of dream interpretation. This method, sometimes referred to as "tangential thinking" opens a new avenue of understanding for nurses through which the content of communications with patients may reveal crucial emotional needs of patients or nurses that otherwise remain hidden.

Symbols are modes of expression common to science, art, literature, dance, education, religion, and all other areas of life; they are not something special but are conventional, general, or accidental in nature. There are not three distinct types; there is a continuum from one type to another. Some of the symbols in the central range seem to be universally used; some are culturally conditioned; some are highly personal or autistic. Works of art, myths, dreams, and other symbolic expressions that are nonrational can be understood when the feelings and underlying insights that they express become known.

Nonrational expressions are particular kinds of perceptions in which inner experiences are perceived as though they came through sensory channels, from objects outside the self.[33] Dreams, for example, are expressions of felt difficulties that appear under the conditions of sleep. While dreams may be analyzed and interpreted, nurses require consistent assistance from individuals competent in aiding them in this educating procedure. The basis for interpretation and its importance is here cited so that nurses may deal more intelligently with various misconceptions and superstitions concerning dreams and dream interpretation. Likewise, they are suggested as a challenge to nurses for developing skill in identifying cues in communications from patients that tell nurses more than the patient can reveal directly.

For example, the following "prophetic dream" may be

[33] Erich Fromm, *The Forgotten Language* (New York, Rinehart & Co., Inc., 1951). Ch. II, pp. 11-23.

cited: A patient, multipara IV, presented herself at a maternity clinic in the sixth month with evidence of uterine bleeding. On inspection polyps were discovered. A specimen was obtained for further laboratory examination and the patient's husband informed of the possibility of a finding of malignancy. The patient was hospitalized for observation and treatment, pending the report. Meanwhile, the husband returned home to make plans for the other three children. One may assume that there was manifest anxiety concerning the outcome of laboratory reports, and the possible outcomes for his wife, and for the care of children already born. In addition, the religious affiliations of the husband and patient prevented them from readily considering the possibility of surgical intervention, in order to save the life of the patient as opposed to that of the child, if this eventuality became necessary. On the basis of these events, the patient's husband retired to bed that night where, under the conditions of sleep, he had the following dream:

"I dreamed that my wife was on the operating table and the surgeon was about to operate; he had the knife in his hand. I rushed in and shouted, 'Don't operate, I can't give my permission.' Whereupon the surgeon dropped the knife and remarked, 'Oh, all right, she doesn't have cancer anyway.' "

The wish for personal power and ability to intervene, to bring about a happy ending to the present dilemma and the critical conflicts it generated are inherent in the dream. Coincidently, the laboratory reported "negative findings"; husband, patient, other patients, nurses, and doctors were considerably impressed with the prophecy inherent in the dream. Actually, the facts on which the prophecy is based were all available to the husband, who, under conditions of sleep, selected those factors available to him that were in line with his real and positive feelings toward his wife, as well as the ethical conceptions he preferred to follow. If his character has been such as to select more hostile elements he might have dreamed that his wife had cancer and that she died. The main theme in the dream is: I wish I had power to stop the whole process and end the problem. For reasons unknown he cannot express these feelings directly and uses the dream to convey his powerlessness in the situation.

Fromm asserts that the themes in a dream are significant, expressing profound insights about the self. The dreamer is always in the dream; it arises from and through his concern for self. Dreams are always specific and show wishes, longings and desires not recognized by the dreamer in waking life.

For example, a child in a hospital situation dreamed: I was in a boat; there were two of us. I knew that the boat would sink and then a terrible storm came up. I was afraid. I knew if I held up the part where the sail was that the boat would not sink and I did and we got into the shore." Many feelings are shown in this dream and the need to make personal effort in a situation that became stormy is indicated; this is actually what the child's later behavior indicated although she never verbalized this need directly and forgot the dream soon after telling it to the nurse.

Understanding the method of dream interpretation, and the dynamics of symbolization, makes it possible for nurses to recognize more deeply the meaning of defenses for managing anxiety in communications with patients. It opens an area of communication with others beyond that expressed in spoken language. Occasionally critical cues to destructive, suicidal wishes are inherent in nonrational communications such as poems about death, depressions, or pictures that show figures who have fallen out of a window. Often, nonrational expressions are cues that a nurse can pick up and use for her own purposes; interpreting them to patients is not indicated. Often she may avert serious tragedy for the family of a patient who shows a suicidal tendency.

The body as a whole, as well as parts of it, act as expressional instruments that communicate to others the feelings, wishes, and aspirations of an individual. Like speech; attitudes, dreams, folk songs, gestures, and the like are expressive and communicative acts. They are productions that are individual and cultural and signify a stage of development in ability to communicate. Gestures of the body, or the form in which posture or movement expresses feelings, represent a kind of communication that symbolizes at once the goal of the movement as well as the manner in which achievement of it will occur. This principle is perhaps best revealed in the posture of the extremely "regressed" patient whose catatonic posture indicates his wish for a relationship as warm, comforting, and protective as intrauterine existence and the psychological dependence it implies. The gesture, like verbal behavior, is a way of translating inner perceptions, thoughts, and meanings of experience into participation in life; both are dependent upon feelings and are ways of giving form to their expression.

At first, body gestures are spontaneous expressions of feelings as perceived; the newborn infant, for example shows random behavior when his feelings of well-being are disturbed by loss of support; there is a gross, mass response that is poorly organized and unproductive. Gradually, gestures connected with specific events become formalized in conventional ways. Conventional gestures may gain universal meaning in a particular culture, examples being tipping the hat, waving good-by, kneeling for prayer, and the like. These may be distinguished, for purposes of study of human behavior, from more individualized gestures which express intensities of feelings and kinds of thought that are specific in certain situations and are expressed in individual ways through a particular constitutional endowment. Thus they give form to the expression of personality through bodily movement.

Gestures may involve the whole body, as may be seen in total responses referred to as "underactivity" or "overactivity" of patients. The total organism enters into the expression of anxiety and emotionalized feelings either through the total inhibition or overchannelization of overt expression of anxiety or through the random behavior when energy is not specifically channeled. Gestures may be substitutive expressions for verbalizations of positive feelings, as was the V sign, indicating faith in victory during World War II. They may be substitutive for feelings connected with anxiety, such as hostility and resentment that cannot be expressed directly, verbally. Such intent is often implicit in facial grimaces that are menacing, biting of lips, continual clearing of the throat, sniffing inappropriately, and the like. Other behavior not directly connected with active participation in an event but that indicates the wish to avoid such participation and to hide the feelings that are opposite to those shared in the ongoing activity, includes doodling, toying with cigarettes and pencils, stroking the hands through the hairs, etc. These out-of-field behaviors or gestures express wishes, longings, resentments and may function as cues to others that there are feelings that cannot be openly revealed in the situation. Symonds makes reference to gestures as symbolic of feelings of hostility performed in abbreviated acts, such as mannerisms and tics, that serve to annoy others without risking possible counteraggression.[34]

The nurse's gestures in relations with patients show how she feels about a particular patient or some aspect of his care. Patients often use various body parts to symbolize their feelings that cannot be expressed directly; a headache might imply "something in my situation is giving me a pain in the head." Loss of sensation in an extremity might mean, "I don't perceive or feel anything that I come into contact with." These observations in patients are always hunches about the meaning of the way in which a patient expresses a felt difficulty and may be ruled out on further organic evidence. They provide clues to interpersonal difficulties, problems the patient faces in relations with others. A nurse might experience dysmenorrhea; it might mean defective uterine position and it might mean, "This business of being a woman gives me a pain in the belly."

Interpretations of nonrational communications, through dreams or words used to express a difficulty, or through use of a body part, are always held contingent upon further evidence of the wishes, longings, hostility, or resentment that may be

[34] Symonds, *op. cit.*, p. 472.

involved in the expression. In literature on psychosomatic medicine a considerable amount of evidence is being gathered to support the conception that there is an emotional basis for many of the difficulties expressed in relations with patients in general hospitals.

Recording

In relations with patients nurses can attend precisely to the way in which a difficulty is stated by the patient. The exact wording is more important than abbreviated or cryptic recording of the complaint. For example, charting "the patient complains of backache" is one note; recording what the patient says, for example, "I have a pain in the back of me," may have considerable more significance when all physical findings are negative. Is the patient saying, in effect, "Something in my past still hurts, and I'm saying it through my back"?

Forms for recording data grow out of specific studies that are under way. While student nurses are expected to record on charts of patients, and their contribution is a valuable one in many respects, their view of the purposes and usefulness of recording can be constricted when charting on specific hospital forms is the only recorded contribution required of them. As students are asked to study interaction in relations with patients new forms will be required: students will develop these forms themselves in order to record particular kinds of data they are gathering. When observational standpoints and units for observation, hypotheses to be studied, are included in the method used to aid students to develop skill in observation they will merit charts that are different from the usual ones.

Developing a form that will simplify recording relations and techniques for making studies that contribute to clinical research in nursing requires initiative. Alertness to what a nurse sees on her own, without prodding from others, grows as she is faced with the responsibility of thinking through the steps in a study of her relations with a patient and the best ways in which she can organize her data for analysis and for communicating it to others.

A simple form that has been found useful in aiding nurses to become aware of their feelings in relations with patients

FORM #1   NURSING PROCESS STUDY

Step #1. Using random or spectator observation of a patient, record what is observed about the patient and state an hypothesis to be studied. You may want to use your first contact for this purpose.

Step #2. State your hypothesis and show how you plan to study your relations with the patient in order to test it. Make an appointment for conference time if you wish.

Step #3. Using participant observation, make a cross-sectional study of all observations over the period of time as decided upon in class by the student group. Use the following form

Page #1.   Page #2.

Responses of the patient:	Responses of the nurse:	Analysis and speculations by the nurse.	Comments by the . instructor; leave blank for conference later.
Step A. Record observations of the patient as you approached him.			
	Step B. Record your opening remarks, your feelings and thoughts about the patient.		
Step C. Record the patient's responses to your remarks and attitudes.		—Scotch tape here—	
	Step D. Record your responses.		
Step E. Continue this process for as long a period of time as has been decided upon. Try to record accurately every detail of what transpires including feelings, gestures, materials offered to patient, the mood and manner of offering them, etc. You may wish to make your notes in the presence of the patient; your purpose must be clarified with him. You may make your notes afterward from memory if the patient objects to your writing down what is said.			

Step #4. Transfer your data to sheets of paper ruled in two columns, as indicated above. Put the finished report away for a few days before proceeding to step #5.

Step #5. Analyze your data in the light of your hypothesis, or in terms of needs expressed, energy transformed into recurring or unique patterns of action, or in the light of subject matter discussed in class, or what happened in this relationship as you see it. Use scotch tape to attach page #2, the analysis sheet, so that it can be compared point by point with your data.

Step #6. Arrange for a one-hour conference with the instructor to discuss your findings.

Fig. 17.   A form for recording relations in nursing.

and in gathering data that can later be studied with greater objectivity than is possible during a first attempt in studying interpersonal relations is suggested in Fig. 17, p. 308. Many students who have used this form have found it difficult, initially, to write down their own behavior in a situation. However, once these students struggled through this difficulty they found that initial insights into their own behavior and into the ways in which patients responded to them expanded rather rapidly. Most students who have used this form have verified the principle that *changes in the behavior of patients is largely dependent upon changes in the behavior of the nurse in the situation with them.*

Summary

Observation, communication, and recording are all interlocking performances in interpersonal relations that make it possible for nurses to study what is happening in their contacts with patients. Methods discussed in this chapter are ones considered valuable to the use of nursing as an interpersonal process that is therapeutic and educative for patients. Other methods are offered in literature well known to nurses. Nurses observe the ways in which patients transform energy into patterns of action that bring satisfaction or security in the face of a recurring problem. Nurses and patients communicate with one another in terms of their views of themselves and their expectations of others. When the difficulties of patients are recorded in verbatim accounts they can often be desymbolized to reveal hidden wishes and longings that are often, but not always, the root of the problem they are facing at a given period in time. Studying nursing as an interpersonal process calls for the development of novel forms that meet the student nurse's requirements; data gathered in studies other than that recorded on charts may serve as a real contribution to the understanding of interpersonal conditions that are required for health. One form that has been used in nursing is suggested.

Selected Bibliography (by topics)

Anxiety

Anxiety, Paul Hoch, ed. New York: Grune & Stratton, Inc., 1950.

Cannon, Walter B. *Bodily Changes in Pain, Hunger, Fear and Rage*. New York: Appleton-Century-Crofts, Inc., 1927.

Freud, Sigmund. *The Problem of Anxiety*. New York: W. W. Norton & Company, Inc., 1936.

Gittelson, M. "The Role of Anxiety in Somatic Disease." *Annals of Internal Medicine*, 28:289-97 (February, 1948).

Hartogs, Renatus. "The Clinical Investigation and Differential Measurement of Anxiety." *American Journal of Psychiatry*, 106:929-34 (June, 1950).

Horney, Karen. *Our Inner Conflicts*. New York: W. W. Norton & Company, Inc., 1945.

Klein, H. R., Potter, H. W., and Dyk, R. B. *Anxiety in Pregnancy and Childbirth*. New York: Paul B. Hoeber, Inc., 1950.

May, Rollo. *The Meaning of Anxiety*. New York: The Ronald Press Company, 1950.

Meerloo, Joost A. M. *Patterns of Panic*. New York: International Universities Press, Inc., 1950.

Miller, N. E., and Dollard, John. *Social Learning and Imitation*. New Haven: Yale University Press, 1941.

Mowrer, O. H. "Anxiety Reduction and Learning." *Journal of Experimental Psychology*, 27:497-516 (1940).

See also Footnotes in Chapter 7.

Child Development

Aldrich, C. Anderson. *Babies Are Human Beings*. New York: The Macmillan Company, 1938.

————. *Feeding Our Old-Fashioned Children*. New York: The Macmillan Company, 1941.

Association for Childhood Education. *Healthful Living for Children*. Washington, D.C., 1947.

Bakwin, Harry. *Psychological Care during Infancy and Childhood.* New York: D. Appleton-Century Company, 1944.

Baruch, Dorothy. *New Ways in Discipline.* New York: McGraw-Hill Book Company, 1949.

Beck, Lester F. *Human Growth.* New York: Harcourt, Brace & Company, 1949.

Beverly, Bert I. *A Psychology of Growth.* New York: McGraw-Hill Book Company, 1947.

Blos, Peter. *The Adolescent Personality.* New York: D. Appleton-Century Company, 1941.

Bossard, James H. S. *The Sociology of Child Development.* New York: Harper & Brothers, 1948.

Chaplin, Dora P. *Children and Religion.* New York: Charles Scribner's Sons, 1948.

Jersild, Arthur T. *Child Psychology.* New York: Prentice-Hall, Inc., 1947.

———. *Child Development and the Curriculum.* New York: Columbia University Press, 1946.

Jersild, Arthur, and Tasch, Ruth J. *Children's Interests.* New York: Teachers College Bureau of Publications, 1949.

Sacks, Hilda. *So Your Child Won't Eat.* New York: Robert M. McBride & Company, 1946.

Senn, Milton. *All about Feeding Children.* New York: Doubleday Doran & Company, 1944.

Spock, Benjamin. *The Common Sense Book of Baby and Child Care.* New York: Duell, Sloane & Pearce Co., 1945.

Communication

Chase, Stuart. *The Tyranny of Words.* New York: Harcourt, Brace & Company, Inc., 1938.

Hayakawa, S. I. *Language in Action.* New York: Harcourt, Brace & Company, Inc., 1941.

Johnson, Wendell. *People in Quandaries: The Semantics of Personal Adjustment.* New York: Harper & Brothers, 1946.

Langer, Suzanne K. *Philosophy in a New Key.* Cambridge: Harvard University Press, 1942.

Larrabee, Harold A. *Reliable Knowledge.* Boston: Houghton Mifflin Company, 1945.

Lazarsfeld, Paul F., and Kendall, Patricia. "The Listener Talks Back, Report on a Test of a Public Health Program," in *Radio in Health Education.* New York: Columbia University Press, 1945.

Lee, I. J. *Language Habits in Human Affairs* New York: Harper & Brothers, 1941.

Morris, Charles. *Signs, Language and Behavior.* New York: Prentice-Hall, Inc., 1946.

Murray, E. *The Speech Personality*, rev. ed. Philadelphia: J. B. Lippincott Company, 1944.

Ogden, C. K., and Richards, I. A. *The Meaning of Meaning.* New York: Harcourt, Brace & Company, Inc., 1945.

Sapir, Edward. "Communication," in *Encyclopedia of the Social Sciences.* New York: The Macmillan Company, Vol. 4 (1931), pp. 78-80.

————. "Symbolism," in *Encyclopedia of the Social Sciences.* New York: The Macmillan Company, Vol. 14 (1934), pp. 492-95.

Conflict

Barker, R. G. "An Experimental Study of the Resolution of Conflicts in Children," in McNemar, Quinn & M. A. Merrill, editors, *Studies in Personality.* New York: McGraw-Hill Book Company, Inc., 1942, Ch. II.

Brown, J. S. "Factors Determining Conflict Reactions in Difficult Discriminations." *Journal of Experimental Psychology* (1942), pp. 272-92.

Guthrie, E. R. *The Psychology of Human Conflict.* New York: Harper & Brothers, 1938.

Horney, K. *Our Inner Conflicts.* New York: W. W. Norton & Company, Inc., 1945.

Hovland, C. I., and Sears, R. R. "Experiments on Motor Conflicts, I, Types of Conflicts and Their Modes of Resolution." *Journal of Experimental Psychology*, 23:477-93 (1938).

Lewin, Kurt. *Resolving Social Conflicts.* New York: Harper & Brothers, 1948.

————. *A Dynamic Theory of Personality.* New York: McGraw-Hill Book Company, Inc., 1935.

Luria, A. R. *The Nature of Human Conflict,* trans. by W. H. Gantt. New York: Liveright Publishing Corporation, 1932.

Maslow, A. H. "Conflict, Frustration, and the Theory of Threat." *The Journal of Abnormal and Social Psychology*, 38:81-86 (1943).

Miller, N. E. "Experimental Studies of Conflict," in J. McV. Hunt, ed., *Personality and the Behavior Disorders.* New York: The Ronald Press Company, 1944, Vol. 1, Ch. XIV, pp. 431-65.

————. "Analysis of the Form of Conflict Reactions." *Psychology Bulletin*, 37:720 (1937).

Washburne, J. N. *Social Adjustment Inventory.* Yonkers-on-Hudson, New York: World Book Company, 1940.

Frustration

Bateson, G. "The Frustration-Aggression Hypothesis and Culture," *Psychology*, 48:350-55 (November, 1941).

Dollard, J., Doob, L. W., Miller, N. E., Mowrer, O. H., and Sears, R. R. *Frustration and Aggression.* New Haven: Yale University Press, 1939.

Kardiner, A. *The Individual and His Society.* New York: Columbia University Press, 1939.

Shaffer, L. R. *Psychology of Adjustment.* Boston: Houghton Mifflin Company, 1936.

General Methods

Abt, Lawrence E., and Bellak, Leopold. *Projective Psychology.* New York: Alfred A. Knopf, 1951.

Bingham, W. V. *How to Interview.* New York: Harper & Brothers, 1941.

Carr, Lowell J. *Situational Analysis: An Observational Approach to Introductory Sociology.* New York: Harper & Brothers, 1948.

Garrett, A. *Interviewing: Its Principles and Methods.* New York: Family Welfare Association of America, 1942.

Lippitt, R. *Training in Community Relations: A Research Exploration toward New Group Skills.* New York: Harper & Brothers, 1949.

Preu, Paul W. *Outline of Psychiatric Case Study.* New York: Paul B. Hoeber, Inc., 1943.

Shank, Donald J., *et al. The Teacher as Counselor,* Series VI-Student Personnel Work, pamphlet. Washington, D.C.: American Council on Education, 1948.

Whitehorn, J. "The Art of Interviewing." *Archives of Neurology and Psychiatry,* **52**:197-216 (1944).

Young, Pauline V. *Interviewing in Social Work.* New York: McGraw-Hill Book Company, Inc., 1935.

Guilt

Klein, Melanie, and Riviere, Joan. *Love, Hate and Reparation.* Psychoanalytic Epitomes No. 2. London: Hogarth Press, Ltd., 1937.

Illness, as an Event

Abeles, M. M. "Post-operative Psychoses." *American Journal of Psychiatry,* **94**:1187-1203 (1938).

Anonymous. *The Philosophy of Insanity: By a Late Inmate of the Royal Asylum for Lunatics at Gartnavel.* Glasgow, 1860, reprinted, New York: Greenberg, 1947.

Barton, Betsy. *And So to Live Again.* New York: Appleton-Century-Crofts, Inc., 1944.

Bernays, Edw. L. "What Patients Say about Nursing." *American Journal of Nursing* (February, 1947). Vol. 47.

Boison, Anton T. *The Exploration of the Inner World.* Chicago: Willett, Clark & Company, 1936.

Carlson, E. R. *Born That Way.* New York: John Day Company, 1941.

Day, J. W. "A Patient's View of a Hospital." *Hospitals,* **14**:18-21 (1940).

Harrison, C. Y. *Thank God for My Heart Attack.* New York: Henry Holt & Company, Inc., 1948.

Hathway, Kath. B. *The Little Locksmith.* New York: Coward-McCann, Inc., 1943.

Hoopes, G. *Out of the Running,* Springfield, Illinois: Charles C. Thomas, 1939.

Kahn, E. "Aspects of Normal Personality Experiencing Disease." *Yale Journal of Biology and Medicine* 13:397-408 (1941).

Levy, D. M. "Psychic Trauma of Operations in Children." *American Journal of Diseases of Children,* 69:7-25 (1945).

Plageman, Bentz. *My Place to Stand.* New York: Farrar, Straus & Company, 1949.

Leadership

Adorno, T. W., *et al. The Authoritarian Personality.* New York: Harper & Brothers, 1950.

Jennings, Helen H. *Leadership and Isolation: A Study of Personality in Inter-personal Relations.* New York: Longmans, Green & Company, Inc., 1943.

Redl, Fritz. "Group Emotions and Leadership." *Psychiatry,* 5:573-92 (1942).

Schmidt, Richard. "Leadership," in *Encyclopedia of the Social Sciences.* New York: The Macmillan Company. 9:282-87.

Whitehead, Alfred North. *Leadership in a Free Society.* Cambridge: Harvard University Press, 1936.

Learning

Bateson, G. "Social Planning and the Concept of 'Deutero-learning,'" in T. M. Newcomb and E. L. Hartley (eds.) *Readings in Social Psychology.* New York: Henry Holt & Company, Inc., 1947.

Cantor, Nathaniel. *Dynamics of Learning.* Buffalo, New York: Foster & Stewart Publishing Corporation, 1946.

Guthrie, E. R. *Psychology of Learning.* New York: Harper & Brothers, 1935.

Hilgard, E. R. *Theories of Learning.* New York: Appleton-Century-Crofts, Inc. 1948.

Hilgard, E. R., and Marguis, D. G. *Conditioning and Learning.* New York: Appleton-Century-Crofts, Inc., 1940.

Hull, Clark L. *The Principles of Behavior.* New York: Appleton-Century-Crofts, Inc., 1943.

McGeoch, John A. *The Psychology of Human Learning.* New York: Longmans, Green & Company, Inc., 1942.

Mowrer, O. Hobart. *Learning Theory and Personality Dynamics.* New York: The Ronald Press Company, 1950.

Murphy, Lois, and Ladd, Henry. *Emotional Factors in Learning.* New York: Columbia University Press, 1944.

Muse, Maude B. *Guiding Learning Experience.* New York: The Macmillan Company, 1950.

Tolman, Edward C. *Purposive Behavior in Animals and Men.* New York: Appleton-Century-Crofts, Inc., 1932.

White, Ralph K. "The Case for the Tolman-Lewin Interpretations of Learning." *Psychological Review,* 50:157-86 (1943).

Motivation

Hawley, Paul R. "The Role of Motivation in Recovery from Illness." *American Journal of Psychiatry,* Vol. 104, No. 12 (June, 1948).

Kubie, L. S. "Motivation and Rehabilitation." *Psychiatry,* 8:69-78 (1945).

Linton, Ralph. *The Cultural Background of Personality.* New York: Appleton-Century-Crofts, Inc., 1945.

Sherif, M., and Cantril, H. *The Psychology of Ego-Involvements.* New York: John Wiley & Sons, Inc., 1947.

Needs

Cannon, W. B. *The Wisdom of the Body.* New York: W. W. Norton & Company, 1939.

————. "Hunger and Thirst," in Carl Murchinson, ed. *A Handbook of General Experimental Psychology.* Worcester: Clark University Press, 1934, Ch. V.

Murray, H. A., *et al. Exploration in Personality.* New York: Oxford University Press, 1938.

Ribble, Margaret. "Infantile Experience in Relation to Personality Development," in J. McV. Hunt, ed. *Personality and the Behavior Disorder,* Vol. II, Ch. XX, pp. 621-51.

Skard, A. G. "Needs and Need Energy." *Character and Personality,* 8:28-41 (1939).

Parental Roles

Anshen, Ruth Nanda, ed. *The Family: Its Function and Destiny.* New York: Harper & Brothers, 1949.

Baruch, D. W. *Parents Can Be People: A Primer for and about Parents.* New York: Appleton-Century-Crofts, Inc., 1944.

————. *New Ways in Discipline.* New York: McGraw-Hill Book Company, Inc., 1949.

Bently, Madison. "Who Is to Bear Primary Responsibility for the Psychological Disorders." *American Journal of Psychology,* Vol. LXII, No. 2 (April, 1949), p. 257.

Deutsch, H. *Psychology of Women; A Psychoanalytic Interpretation:* Vol. I, *Girlhood;* Vol. II, *Motherhood.* New York: Grune & Stratton, Inc., 1945.

Fitzsimmons, Margaret. "Treatment of Problems of Dependency Related to Permanent Physical Handicap." *Family,* 23:329-36 (1943).

Flügel, J. C. *The Psychoanalytic Study of the Family*. London: Hogarth Press, Ltd., 1950.

Fromm-Reichmann, Frieda. *Notes on the Mother Role in the Family Group*. Bulletin of the Menninger Clinic, Vol. 4, No. 5 (September, 1940).

Levy, John, and Munroe, Ruth. *The Happy Family*. New York: Alfred A. Knopf, 1938.

Symonds, P. *The Dynamics of Parent-Child Relationships*. New York: Bureau of Publications, Teachers College, 1949.

Yugend, L. "The Role of Parental Attitudes in the Treatment of Diseases in Children." *Mental Hygiene*, 25:591-605 (1941).

Personality

Cole, Luella. *Psychology of Adolescence*. New York: Rinehart and Company, Inc., 1949.

Erickson, Erik H. *Childhood and Society*. New York: W. W. Norton & Company, 1950.

Fromm, Erich. *Man for Himself*. New York: Rinehart & Company, Inc., 1947.

Josselyn, Irene M. *Psychosexual Development of Children*. Pamphlet, Family Service Association of America, 122 East 22 Street, New York, 10.

Kluckhohn, Clyde, and Murray, H. A. *Personality: In Nature, Society and Culture*. New York: Alfred A. Knopf, 1949.

Lane, Homer. *Talks to Parents and Teachers*. New York: Hermitage House Inc., 1949.

Montagu, Ashley. *On Being Human*. New York: Henry Schuman, Inc., 1950.

Plant, James S. *The Envelop*. New York: Commonwealth Fund, 1950.

Psychopathology

Cameron, N. *The Psychology of Behavior Disorders*. Boston: Houghton Mifflin Company, 1947.

English, O. Spurgeon, and Pearson, Gerald H. J. *Common Neuroses in Children and Adults*. New York: W. W. Norton & Company, Inc., 1937.

Fenichel, O. *Psychoanalytic Theory of Neurosis*. New York: W. W. Norton & Company, Inc., 1945.

Goldstein, Kurt. *Human Nature in the Light of Psychopathology*. Cambridge: Harvard University Press, 1940.

Nielson, J. M. *The Engrammes of Psychiatry*. Springfield, Illinois: Charles C. Thomas, 1947.

Noyes, A. P. *Modern Clinical Psychiatry*. New York: The Macmillan Company, 1948.

Tompkins, Silvan S. *Contemporary Psychopathology*. Cambridge: Harvard University Press, 1943.

Psychosomatic Method

Alexander, Franz. *Psychosomatic Medicine*. New York: W. W. Norton & Company, Inc., 1950.

Dunbar, Flanders. *Synopsis of Psychosomatic Diagnosis and Treatment*. St. Louis: The C. V. Mosby Company, 1948.

Hinsie, Leland E. *The Person in the Body, an Introduction to Psychosomatic Medicine*. New York: W. W. Norton & Company, Inc., 1945.

Strecker, E. A. "Psychosomatics." *Journal of the American Medical Association*, 134:1520-21 (August 30, 1947).

Weiss, Edward, and English, O. S. *Psychosomatic Medicine*. Philadelphia: W. B. Saunders Company, 1943.

Therapeutic Methods

Arthur, Grace. *Tutoring as Therapy*. New York: Commonwealth Fund, 1946.

Alexander, F., and French, T. M. *Psychoanalytic Therapy*. New York: The Ronald Press Company, 1946.

Allen, F. H. *Psychotherapy with Children*. New York: W. W. Norton & Company, Inc., 1942.

"Areas of Agreement in Psychotherapy," a symposium. *American Journal of Orthopsychiatry*, 10:698-709 (1940).

Bettelheim, Bruno. *Love Is Not Enough*. Glencoe, Illinois: Free Press, 1950.

Brenman, M., and Gill, M. M. *Hypnotherapy: A Survey of the Literature*. New York: International Universities Press, 1947.

Davis, J. Eisele. *Rehabilitation: Its Principles & Practice*. New York: A. S. Barnes & Company, Inc., 1946.

Fenichel, O. "Problems of Psychoanalytic Techniques." *Psychoanalytic Quarterly* (1941), 130 pp.

Fromm-Reichmann, Frieda. *Principles of Intensive Psychotherapy*. Chicago: University of Chicago Press, 1950.

Grunker, R. R., and Spiegel, J. E. *Men Under Stress*. Philadelphia: The Blakiston Company, 1945.

Hamilton, Gordon. *Psychotherapy in Child Guidance*. New York: Columbia University Press, 1947.

Herzberg, A. *Active Psychotherapy*. New York: Grune & Stratton, Inc., 1945.

Hinsie, Leland B. *Concepts and Problems of Psychotherapy*. New York: Columbia University Press, 1937.

Klein, Melanie. *The Psychoanalysis of Children*. London: Hogarth Press, Ltd., 1932.

Knight, R. P. "Evaluation of the Results of Psychoanalytic Therapy." *American Journal of Psychiatry*, 98:434-46 (1941).

Law, Stanley G. *Therapy Through Interview*. New York: McGraw-Hill Book Company, Inc., 1948.

Lecky, Prescott. *Self-Consistency.* New York: Island Press Coop., Inc., 1945.

Levine, Maurice. *Psychotherapy in Medical Practice.* New York: The Macmillan Company, 1942.

Lorand, Sandor. *The Technique of Psychoanalytic Therapy.* New York: International Universities Press, 1945.

Moore, Dom T. *Nature and Treatment of Mental Disorders.* New York: Grune & Stratton, Inc., 1943.

Moreno, J. L. "Psychodramatic Shock Therapy." *Sociometry,* 2:1-30 (1931).

Rogers, C. R. *Counseling and Psychotherapy.* Boston: Houghton Mifflin Company, 1942.

Rosenzweig, Saul. *Psychodiagnostics.* New York: Grune & Stratton, Inc., 1949.

————. "Some Implicit Common Factors in Diverse Methods of Psychotherapy." *American Journal of Orthopsychiatry,* 6:412-15 (1936).

Schilder, Paul. *Psychotherapy.* New York: W. W. Norton & Company, Inc., 1938.

Smith, Geddes. *Psychotherapy in General Medicine.* New York: The Commonwealth Fund, 1946.

Sullivan, H. S. *Conceptions of Modern Psychiatry.* Washington, D.C.: William Alanson White Psychiatric Foundation, 1947.

Taft, Jessie. "The Dynamics of Therapy." New York: The Macmillan Company, 1933.

Willoughby, R. R. "An Operational Approach to the Problem of Emotional Readjustment." *The Journal of Abnormal and Social Psychology,* 33:261-64 (1938).

Index

Italics indicate references relative to principles, generalizations, and significant terms and statements.

Pattern of movement, 162
Pediatric nursing, 13
Pediatricians, 250
Pediatrics, 141
Peers, 267
People: avoidance of relations with, *109,
114*; difference between, *53*; philosophy
about, 68; in school of nursing, relating
therapeutically to, 267
Perception, *57*, 156, *163*, *185*, 221; in
communication, 296–97, *302*; functioning of the child in relation to his, *213*;
inner, 305; movement of, 34, 35; narrowing of, *128*
Perpetuation of the species, 79
Person, *52*, *212*, *270*, 272; biting kind of,
232; development of, *141*; disrespect for,
245; feelings of others about the individual as a, *212*; as he is, 154; inability to
accept as a, *234*; interest in, *253*; kind of,
x; productive, 69; professional, *107*;
respect for, *9*, 111, *253*
Personality: building blocks of, 166;
changes in, 131; definition of, 164–65,
271–72; determination of, *163*; development of, x, 37, *57*, 58, 73, 83, 84, 86, 87,
199; distortion of, 167; expansion of,
130, 165, 225; expression of, 167, 223,
305; formation and functioning as influenced by mothering experiences,
216, 217; formation in childhood, 62,
190–98, 210–22; formation in infancy,
162–69; forward movement of, *12, 16*;
function of, 73; hindrance to expression,
53; importance of, x, xi; mobilization of,
223; movement of, 119; organization of,
132–33, 298; psychological experiences
that influence, 35; psychosexual stages
of organization of, 166; raw materials of,
162, 163; reconstruction of, 119, 226;
reorganization of, 93, 133; shaping of,
163; strengthening, *31*, 157; threat to,
27, 87, 93, 113, 132, 136, 234, 241;
understanding, 237
Personality, eras of development: adolescence, 246–47; juvenile era, 241–45;
preadolescence, 245–46
Personifications, 300
Persuasion, 28

Philosophy, 57, 68
Phobias, 146–50, 155; in a child, example
of, 148–49; purposive aspect of, 147
Physician, relationship with, 45
Planning, co-operative, 25
Pleasure, 130, 166, 167
Polar constructs, 126, 299
Policies, *288*
Poliomyelitis, 266
Positive groping, 172
Posture, 305
Poverty, 222
Power, 36, 82, 110, 114, 172, 243, 245;
authoritative, 235; in childhood, assert-
ing, 262; exertion of, 232; individ-
ual, 235; irrational, 235; means, to
strengthen, 207; rational, 235; shifting
of, *40*
Powerlessness, 31, 32, 52, 67, 80, 113, 169,
186, 202, 226, 235; examples of, 255–56,
304; in death, 292
Praise in nursing situations, 235–37, 271
Preadolescence, 245–46
Preconceptions, 36, 37, 70, 124, 132, 157,
206, 225; documented example of, 121–
23; about people from certain social
classes, 255; operation of, *123*
Pregnancy, 133, 134
Prejudices, 93–94
Prestige, 82, 91; through continuity in
communication, 293; cultural, 45; defense of, 124; need for, 140, 285; threat
to, 121, *124*, 129
Pride, 154
Principles, ix, *x*, xii, xiii, *142*; as guides to
action, *142*; translating, into action,
267; using resources to identify, 267
Principles, generalizations, and significant terms and statements, *142*
methods for studying nursing as an
interpersonal process
communication, *290, 297, 302*
observation, *264, 265, 269, 270, 273,
274, 276, 281, 282, 283, 284, 286, 288*
recording, *309*
nursing situations, influences in
human needs, *78, 79–80, 82*
interferences to achievement of goals,
86